MENTALIZATION-BASED TREATMENT FOR CHILDREN

MENTALIZATION-BASED TREATMENT FOR CHILDREN
A TIME-LIMITED APPROACH

NICK MIDGLEY, KARIN ENSINK, KARIN LINDQVIST,
NORKA MALBERG, AND NICOLE MULLER

American Psychological Association • Washington, DC

Published by
American Psychological Association
750 First Street, NE
Washington, DC 20002
www.apa.org

To order
APA Order Department
P.O. Box 92984
Washington, DC 20090-2984
Tel: (800) 374-2721; Direct: (202) 336-5510
Fax: (202) 336-5502; TDD/TTY: (202) 336-6123
Online: www.apa.org/pubs/books
E-mail: order@apa.org

In the U.K., Europe, Africa, and the Middle East, copies may be ordered from
American Psychological Association
3 Henrietta Street
Covent Garden, London
WC2E 8LU England

Typeset in Goudy by Circle Graphics, Inc., Columbia, MD

Printer: Sheridan Books, Chelsea, MI
Cover Designer: Mercury Publishing Services, Inc., Rockville, MD

The opinions and statements published are the responsibility of the authors, and such opinions and statements do not necessarily represent the policies of the American Psychological Association.

Library of Congress Cataloging-in-Publication Data

Names: Midgley, Nick, 1968- author. | Ensink, Karin, author. | Lindqvist, Karin, author. | Malberg, Norka T., author. | Muller, Nicole (Psychotherapist), author. | American Psychological Association, issuing body.
Title: Mentalization-based treatment for children : a time-limited approach / Nick Midgley, Karin Ensink, Karin Lindqvist, Norka Malberg, and Nicole Muller.
Description: First edition. | Washington, DC : American Psychological Association, [2017] | Includes bibliographical references and index.
Identifiers: LCCN 2016045575 | ISBN 9781433827327 | ISBN 1433827328
Subjects: | MESH: Mental Disorders—therapy | Child | Psychotherapy—methods | Theory of Mind | Adolescent
Classification: LCC RJ504 | NLM WS 350.2 | DDC 618.92/8914—dc23
LC record available at https://lccn.loc.gov/2016045575

British Library Cataloguing-in-Publication Data
A CIP record is available from the British Library.

Printed in the United States of America
First Edition

http://dx.doi.org/10.1037/0000028-000

CONTENTS

FOREWORD

PETER FONAGY

It is somewhat paradoxical that the maturity of an approach should have as its marker an extension to the world of children. It is an indicator of the establishment of mentalization-based treatment (MBT) as a therapy that it finds solid and rigorous application in the context of individual child psychotherapy.

MBT is probably not unusual in this regard. The case of "Little Hans" was the reflection of the maturation of Freud's thinking over the first 2 decades of psychoanalysis; behaviorism had its own "Little Albert"; more recently, the extension of cognitive behavioral therapy into therapeutic work with children appeared 15 to 20 years after Aaron Beck's discoveries.

I am, of course, delighted that the exceptionally talented therapeutic group that constructed this treatment guide chose MBT as the framework that, as child clinicians, they felt confident to extend to children and young people, modifying substantially in many places the approach originally manualized and implemented by Anthony Bateman and me for the treatment of personality disorder (MBT–PD). It is heartening that child-focused therapeutic practice can palpably benefit from applying some of the principles that were developed in the context of a treatment approach to personality disorder (Bateman & Fonagy, 2016). The therapeutic techniques have a sense of familiarity and yet are also different; the therapist's stance recommended in MBT–PD to encourage mentalizing is similar to the treatment guide's recommendation for working with children. The similarity is hardly surprising, given the roots of MBT–PD in studies of the development of mentalizing and the grounding of MBT for children (MBT–C) as a developmental intervention. Such differences that arise are linked to the divergent developmental ambitions of the two therapies: MBT–PD tries to free a developed but inhibited or derailed capacity for mentalizing, whereas MBT–C aims to facilitate the developmental process itself, optimizing the environmental conditions necessary for its growth.

Related to the distinction of therapeutic ambitions, there is an important difference in implementation that should be remarked on because it points to a key gap in the arsenal of MBT techniques available for working with adults. MBT–C inevitably entails the collaboration of parents—in this context, in a primarily psychoeducational capacity but also implicitly therapeutically, in the sense of freeing caregivers from inhibitions or distortions of mentalizing in relation to the particular child. The dialectic model of self-development that underpins both approaches suggests that the clarity with which parents see their child as intentional will enhance the child's development of mentalizing (Fonagy, Gergely, & Target, 2007). I wonder whether therapies for adults would be more effective if the key individuals with whom we have effective relationships were recruited to the therapeutic enterprise to support the recovery of balanced mentalizing.

At the heart of the MBT–C approach outlined in this well-constructed manual is the understanding that in each of us, our emerging capacities for envisioning actions in terms of thoughts and feelings crucially depend on the support we are offered by our families and our social networks, which is essential if we are to develop and maintain this stance. The therapist is an obvious partner and during the treatment process will be able to sustain a child's mentalizing and help them experience the value of mentalizing in social relationships and self-recognition. When the therapist is no longer there, children who have not yet recruited peers and adults to help sustain such a contemplative stance will struggle to retain their developmental achievements. The clarity with which this dialectic process is depicted and illustrated by this guide is one of the valuable contributions of Midgley and colleagues' work.

But why is mentalizing important? The authors are eloquent in describing what mentalizing is and how it develops. As developmentalists, they paint a particularly welcome and rich picture of how a child's mind gradually becomes more attuned to the mental world of those around them, especially in the first decade of life. The movement from something intuitive and simply—yet deeply—felt, to a richer awareness of thoughts and feelings, the content of which may be reflected on, empowers social interaction with adults and peers, and generally creates the background for learning about the social world and one's place in it.

Of course, many of these social lessons are painful. Certain experiences, particularly those related to rejection, abandonment, aggression, and persecution, are hard to mentalize and may generate intolerable levels of pain that make the contemplation of mental states of little benefit compared with the risk of hurt that might come from following the thoughts and feelings, ideas and intentions, of a loved but abusive carer or an admired but cruel peer. If a journey is anticipated to be painful, it makes sense not to go on it; some children, perhaps because of biological vulnerabilities or because of social deprivation, will choose not to embark on a voyage around the caregiver's mind or to focus too closely on the thoughts and feelings behind the actions of their friends. Yet these are the essential social contexts from which an understanding of others in mental state terms can be achieved and provide a grounding to self-understanding. The therapist has to be the source of curiosity and excitement that motivates the child to overcome hesitancy toward intersubjective exploration.

Looked at in the way MBT–C frames children's treatment, child psychotherapy is nothing special. It is simply mirroring a natural process of development. This is akin to learning one's first language: Evolution has given us the whole biological toolkit, assuming an appropriate language environment, for acquiring our native tongue. Some children, deprived of appropriate stimulation, struggle to reach their full linguistic potential. The same may be true for mentalization. If there is insufficient interest in the child's agentiveness, certain basic biological processes may not be triggered. Perhaps the child takes the lack of interest as a signal, honed by evolution, to indicate that the social environment is not conducive to prioritizing subjectivity over a challenging physical world.

MBT–C may be most appropriate for children who are attempting to acquire and then master this most human of developmental capacities but whose exploration has been brought to a halt by the challenges the emerging capacity creates: understanding human motivation "in the raw" without sufficient armor to withstand its most threatening implications. The vulnerability may be biological and identify children with insufficient natural resources (e.g., affect regulation) to protect themselves from the implications of discovering malevolence and hostility around them. Their emotional response, however, in turn undermines their capacity for understanding and leaves them increasingly vulnerable to misapprehending the intentions and beliefs of others. Thus, neither biology nor social context in and of itself is sufficient cause; the failure of mentalizing is the failure of "mind in body."

MBT–C is particularly helpful in disrupting the unfortunate pattern of parent-blaming that is evident among some psychotherapists. The intersubjective nature of mentalizing—the idea that we all find our own mind in someone else's thoughts and feelings about us—spreads responsibility across the parent–child dyad. If children hide their mind from parents (again, for either biological or experiential reasons), parents will fail in mentalizing but cannot in any sense be considered at fault; yet parents' limited understanding of their children will place the children at a disadvantage in not being able to learn about themselves because they do not feel understood by their parents. Children make a massive contribution to determining the quality of their environment, and parents of children with a predisposition to hide their mind, to be "difficult" and "unavailable," need support and help if the vicious cycle of an unmentalized relationship is to be avoided. Children need to make their mind available; parents need to be there to take an interest in the child's mind for the child to internalize parents' appreciation and use it to develop a relatively self-sustaining capacity.

The relationship, although transactional, is not one of two equals. The parent is there to "teach" the child. Parenting has the function of setting up the child for a lifetime of social learning. By this, we do not mean learning in school, although some learning (not a lot) also takes place there. In our social contexts, we are constantly learning about how and what to do about the knowledge that is embodied in our culture, about ourselves, and about our relationships and what we may expect of them. This learning has to be selective because not everyone can be trusted. So how do we know who can be? Mentalizing, we believe, is critical in identifying people who have our interests in mind (Fonagy, Luyten, & Allison, 2015). Those who we feel respond to us—to our thoughts and feelings, not just to our behavior—can probably be trusted. With those who neglect us, or misread our minds, we had better remain vigilant.

Poor mentalizing makes it harder to distinguish those who can be trusted from those who cannot. It undermines the process of social learning. This is perhaps the most important justification for a guide to implement an MBT approach for children: They have so much to learn. If learning in general is undermined by profound difficulties in mentalizing because the source of knowledge is not self-evidently trustworthy, then a mentalization-based approach may be the most helpful and important thing that we can provide. It can enable children to access and benefit from the wealth of knowledge they are primed to acquire from teachers (in the form of any adult) as part of their socialization into the world in which they live. So although this treatment guide is focused on treating children with mental health problems, the mission to improve the quality of mentalizing of our children is to help improve their adaptation to a highly complex social world.

This book is a tremendous achievement, and a highly readable one to boot. It is an essential guide to implementing a treatment approach that is designed to combine therapy with secondary prevention. It is also a guide to enhancing therapeutic work with children inspired by other theoretical orientations. It will be a valuable addition to any clinician's practice library.

ACKNOWLEDGMENTS

We thank the editorial team at the American Psychological Association (APA), especially Susan Reynolds and Ida Audeh, for steering this book through from conception to publication so expertly. The two anonymous reviewers of the manuscript made a range of helpful suggestions, which helped us to "see ourselves from the outside" and modify the text with our readers' needs held better in mind.

We thank the many talented individuals who have contributed to the development of mentalization-based treatment (MBT), especially Peter Fonagy, whose contribution is reflected in the huge number of references we have made to his work and who generously wrote the foreword.

We thank all the families with whom we have worked, who shared their pain, trust, and hopefulness in the context of this work, and especially to the children and families who gave their permission for us to use their images in the book, helping to bring the clinical vignettes to life. The photographs of calendars are taken from children seen at De Jutters Child and Adolescent Mental Health Service (CAMHS) clinic in the Netherlands and are reproduced with permission. The painting in Chapter 6 by Ruth Zuilhof was created especially for this book.

Karin Ensink thanks Peter Fonagy and Mary Target for giving her the opportunity to learn about the development and assessment of mentalization in children. She also thanks Lina Normandin for many years of collaboration and elaborating clinical research and interventions focusing on mentalization in children and parents, especially in the context of trauma.

Karin Lindqvist thanks the Erica Foundation in Stockholm and especially the members of the MBT for children (MBT–C) team, including Jan-Olov Karlsson, Anders Schiöler, and Helena Vesterlund, as well as Agneta Thorén for her contributions to research on MBT–C.

Norka Malberg thanks the members of the New Haven MBT study group and her young child psychiatry seminar members at Yale Child Study Center for their insights and contributions to the evolution of her thinking and clinical practice. Also, thanks to the many families who have helped to shape this work.

Nick Midgley thanks his colleagues (and former colleagues) in the MBT for families (MBT–F) team at the Anna Freud National Centre for Children and Families, including Eia Asen, Dickon Bevington, Helen Brasnett, Jane Dutton, Emma Keaveny, Cathy Troupp, and Sally Wood. Thanks also to the staff at the Crystal Café for keeping him caffeinated while working on the manuscript!

Nicole Muller thanks the De Jutters CAMHS clinic and her MBT team, including Anja van Roon, Debby van Riel, Ruth Zuilhof, Hiske Wolters, Annemarie Boevé, Hanneke Nederhof, and Miranda van der Krans; her supervisees, especially Merlijn Rutten; and Lidewij Gerits, with whom she has taught about MBT–C for many years in an inspiring way.

A version of Chapter 4 was first delivered as a lecture by Nick Midgley, "The Mentalizing Stance in Working With Children," at the KJF Symposium, Lucerne, Switzerland, in 2015. Thanks to Roland Muller, who organized the symposium and gave helpful feedback.

An earlier version of Chapter 5 was first published as an article by Nicole Muller and Nick Midgley, "Approaches to Assessment in Time-Limited Mentalization-Based Therapy for Children (MBT–C)," in *Frontiers in Psychology* (2015) and is reproduced here with thanks to the publishers.

MENTALIZATION-BASED TREATMENT FOR CHILDREN

INTRODUCTION

It has been estimated that at any one time, approximately one in 10 children aged 5 to 16 years suffers from a psychological disorder (Green, McGinnity, Meltzer, Ford, & Goodman, 2005). Among the most common mental health difficulties in children are conduct problems, antisocial behavior, attention-deficit/hyperactivity disorder, depression, and anxiety; emotional disorders are more common in girls, and behavioral problems in boys. As Hagell and Maughan (in press) have pointed out, such mental health problems "have important implications for every aspect of young people's lives including their ability to engage with education, make and keep friends, engage in constructive family relationships and find their own way in the world." We suggest that these problems therefore have important implications for family members, friends, schools, and the wider society.

Although there is now a great variety of evidence-based treatments for children and families, a significant proportion of children still either drop

http://dx.doi.org/10.1037/0000028-001
Mentalization-Based Treatment for Children: A Time-Limited Approach, by N. Midgley, K. Ensink, K. Lindqvist, N. Malberg, and N. Muller

out of therapy or are unable to make use of the available treatments (Fonagy, Luyten, & Allison, 2015). Moreover, many of the evidence-based treatments have been developed for specific populations, making it unrealistic for child therapists to be trained in numerous treatment models relevant to the diverse presenting problems that may bring children to child mental health services. Paradoxically, faced with the wide array of manualized therapies for specific childhood disorders, an increasingly narrow range of approaches is actually made available to children and families, with many child mental health services primarily offering interventions based on a cognitive behavioral therapy (CBT) approach.

Although CBT has a good evidence base for a variety of childhood disorders (McLaughlin, Holliday, Clarke, & Ilie, 2013), and has clearly benefitted many children and families, a one-size-fits-all approach is always dangerous, especially when the evidence suggests that client choice and preference should be at the heart of all good clinical practice. Moreover, many practitioners have experienced situations in which parents and children have difficulties using the kind of strategies that may be offered to manage their problems more effectively, often because they do not have the affect regulation skills or the capacity to make use of the guidance that is a prerequisite for benefitting from such therapeutic approaches (e.g., Scott & Dadds, 2009). We therefore hope that the approach described in this book fills an important gap by offering a short-term, focused intervention for school-age children that draws on traditional psychodynamic principles but integrates them into attachment theory, the empirical study of mentalization, and features of other evidence-based approaches.

OUR APPROACH

In their preface to the *Handbook of Mentalization-Based Treatment*, Allen and Fonagy (2006) wrote,

> In advocating mentalization-based treatment we claim no innovation. On the contrary, mentalization-based treatment is the least novel therapeutic approach imaginable: it addresses the bedrock human capacity to apprehend mind as such. Holding mind in mind is as ancient as human relatedness and self-awareness. (p. xix)

Although this statement might be seen as somewhat disingenuous, there is no doubt that much of what has been described as "mentalization-based treatment" (MBT) will be familiar to therapists coming from different backgrounds—perhaps especially those, like ourselves, who have trained in the psychodynamic tradition. At the same time, we believe that some new ideas have crept in, whether deliberately or accidentally. When running MBT training at the Anna Freud National Centre for Children and Families in London, Dickon Bevington added a typically playful addendum to Allen and Fonagy's (2006) statement, warning that "this product may contain traces of originality. These are only trace contaminants, occurring as part of the production process, and should not spoil your enjoyment of the product" (Asen et al., 2011).

In this book, we describe an approach to working with children therapeutically in a time-limited way that we hope will be both familiar and commonsensical, while offering clinicians a few "traces of originality" that we hope will add something of value to the child therapist's toolbox. We describe the work as a treatment guide because we set out a particular model of treatment, but one that can be adapted and fit to the local contexts in which therapists are working and can be flexible enough to be of use when working with children who present with a range of difficulties.

By focusing on a core capacity that may promote resilience in children with a variety of presenting problems, MBT for children (MBT–C) aims to be a generic therapy that can be adapted to the particular needs of children in middle childhood—roughly ages 5 to 12 years. MBT–C as described in this book is a time-limited, focused intervention that can be easily integrated and used alongside various psychosocial treatments. The overall aim of MBT–C is to promote mentalizing and resilience in such a way that a developmental process is put back on track, and the family and child feel they are better equipped to tackle the problems that first brought them to therapy. Thus, MBT–C aims to both increase the child's capacity for emotional regulation and support parents to best meet the emotional needs of their children.

The basic MBT–C time-limited model is 12 individual sessions, with separate meetings for the parent(s). Although some therapists may view short-term and time-limited therapies as a "necessary evil" in the era of managed care (Salyer, 2002), a significant body of research now suggests that short-term interventions in child mental health can be effective (McLaughlin et al., 2013), including short-term psychodynamic interventions (Abbass, Rabung, Leichsenring, Refseth, & Midgley, 2013). Likewise, a meta-analysis of attachment-focused interventions by Bakermans-Kranenburg, van IJzendoorn, and Juffer (2003) showed that most effective interventions used a moderate number of sessions (between five and 16) and tend to be more focused in their aims.

Time-limited work, when effective, is clearly in the interests of children and families because it allows children to return to their daily lives without too great a disruption to their everyday lives. Nevertheless, there are some children for whom a brief intervention may not be indicated (Ramchandani & Jones, 2003). In certain cases in which a longer term intervention is appropriate (e.g., for those children whose early relational trauma or attachment insecurity makes trusting an adult a real challenge), it is possible to offer up to three blocks of 12 MBT–C sessions (i.e., up to a maximum of 36 sessions). These additional blocks of treatment are based on a review process that weighs the pros and cons of additional treatment, and in these cases, the treatment is never open-ended but continues to be time-limited, with a clear focus and aims.

Like all mentalization-based interventions, the fundamental aim of MBT–C is to enhance skills in mentalizing, both in the parent and the child. For both parents and children, this would include opportunities to practice good mentalizing but also to pay attention to the places where mentalizing breaks down or work on areas where there are deficits in the capacity to mentalize. Such a focus is justified by the fact that research is increasingly demonstrating that the capacity to mentalize contributes to a positive sense of self, healthy relationships, and better emotional regulation (Ensink, Bégin, Normandin, & Fonagy, 2016; Ensink, Berthelot, Bernazzani, Normandin, & Fonagy, 2014). Targeting such capacities is likely to be of value to children (and their parents) with diverse presenting problems, even if the underlying mental health disorder is not "caused" by a failure of mentalization.

As the preceding description implies, the focus of MBT–C is more on process than on content: The aim is not primarily for either parent or child to gain insight into his or her difficulties or to develop an understanding of where these difficulties may have come from; rather, it is to enhance their capacity to use their mentalizing capacity to manage emotions and relationships and to increase the child's capacity to make use of relationships for emotional learning. As such, the ultimate aim of MBT–C is to help the child to make better use of helping relationships after the therapy has ended and for the parents to be better equipped to support their child's development outside and beyond therapy.

ORIGINS OF TIME-LIMITED MBT–C

Although it is not possible to do justice to the rich history of the clinical thinking that has inspired this book, here we briefly sketch out some of the developments that have contributed to this work, and in particular those ideas that have personally informed the authors of this treatment guide.

In Fonagy's 1991 paper, which set out a new way of thinking about borderline states of mind in adults, he referred to "the achievement of a representation of mental events," which he noted had been referred to in the psychoanalytic literature as the *capacity for symbolization*. This term, he suggested, had become "over-burdened with meanings, particularly in psychoanalysis" (p. 641). So he proposed: "For the sake of brevity I would like to label the capacity to conceive of conscious and unconscious mental states in oneself and others as the capacity to *mentalize*" (p. 641, italics in original).

What began as a term used for "the sake of brevity" has taken off in a spectacular fashion in the years since those words were written. In a 2013 review paper about MBT (Bateman & Fonagy, 2013), the authors noted with evident pride that the use of the term *mentalizing* in titles and abstracts of scientific papers on the Web of Science increased from 10 in 1991 to 2,750 in 2011, with numerous authors now using the term, "from psychoanalysts to neuroscientists, from child development researchers to geneticists, from existential philosophers to phenomenologists" (p. 595).

Fonagy's 1991 paper situates the development of the concept of mentalizing at the interface of a number of domains, including research on theory of mind (Premack & Woodruff, 1978) and attachment and reflective functioning (Fonagy, Steele, Steele, Moran, & Higgitt, 1991). But first and foremost, it was a development in the clinical sphere and, in particular, in a way of approaching the treatment of borderline personality disorder (BPD), which Fonagy and Bateman came to reconceptualize as "a disorder of mentalizing" (Bateman & Fonagy, 2010). From the early 1990s, Bateman and Fonagy began to describe certain modifications to the technique of psychodynamic therapy that would follow from a focus on the capacity to mentalize, leading them to propose a new model of therapy for adults with BPD: MBT (Bateman & Fonagy, 2004).

Although MBT was originally developed as a treatment for adults with BPD, in recent years, MBT has been modified for work with children and families (Midgley & Vrouva, 2012). One of the first such developments was short-term mentalization and relational therapy (SMART; Fearon et al., 2006), a family-based intervention later renamed MBT–F (Asen & Fonagy, 2012a, 2012b), which preliminary evaluation has suggested can be helpful for children with a broad range of presenting problems, both internalizing and externalizing (Keaveny et al., 2012). In terms of individual therapy with children, Fonagy and Target's (1996a) model of psychodynamic developmental therapy was perhaps the first treatment approach to be explicitly influenced by emerging ideas about mentalization. A decade later, Verheugt-Pleiter, Zevalkink, and Schmeets (2008) reinterpreted Anne Hurry's (1998) model of psychoanalytic developmental psychotherapy from a mentalization perspective, setting out a model of open-ended therapy that they later described as mentalization-informed child psychoanalytic psychotherapy (Zevalkink, Verheugt-Pleiter, & Fonagy, 2012). As in the work presented here, this approach moves beyond the traditional psychoanalytic approach based on interpretation and developing insight and recognizes that the child therapist is not only a "transference object" but also a "development object"

(A. Freud, 1965), helping to foster new capacities, including improved affect regulation and reflective functioning. Likewise, Ensink and Normandin (2011) elaborated an MBT for sexually abused children, incorporating child psychotherapy techniques developed by Paulina Kernberg (e.g., Kernberg & Chazan, 1991; Kernberg, Weiner, & Bardenstein, 2000), and similar models have been described in case studies by Ramires, Schwan, and Midgley (2012) and Perepletchikova and Goodman (2014). All of these approaches have been open-ended or longer term interventions, often targeted at children with severe histories of neglect and maltreatment and explicitly integrating mentalizing approaches with psychodynamic child therapy.

Developments in MBT have also taken place for both younger and older children. A number of teams have developed mentalization-based interventions with parents and infants (e.g., Etezady & Davis, 2012; Ordway et al., 2014; Slade, Sadler, et al., 2005) and adolescents (e.g., Bleiberg, 2013; Fuggle et al., 2015; Malberg & Fonagy, 2012; Rossouw & Fonagy, 2012; Sharp et al., 2009). Studies have demonstrated the value of mentalization-promoting interventions in school settings (Twemlow, Fonagy, & Sacco, 2005) and school-based psychoeducation programs (Bak, 2012; Bak, Midgley, Zhu, Wistoft, & Obel, 2015). Empirical studies examining what therapists actually do in the consulting room (looking beyond the brand name of therapy) have demonstrated how promoting mentalizing is a feature of psychodynamic therapy and CBT with children, as well as play therapy (Goodman, Midgley, & Schneider, 2016; Goodman, Reed, & Athey-Lloyd, 2015; Muñoz Specht, Ensink, Normandin, & Midgley, 2016). Given the links among attachment, trauma, and mentalizing (see Chapter 2, this volume), it is not surprising that a number of interesting developments have also taken place exploring how ideas about mentalizing can helpfully inform work with children in the context of fostering and adoption (e.g., Bammens, Adkins, & Badger, 2015; Jacobsen, Ha, & Sharp, 2015; Midgley et al., 2017; Muller, Gerits, & Siecker, 2012; Taylor, 2012).

The idea for developing a time-limited model of MBT for school-age children originated at a meeting in London in 2011, which brought together clinicians who were interested in thinking about clinical developments of MBT for children and families. Several members of that group met again in London in the following year, and for a third time in Stockholm in 2013. Working closely with colleagues in this group was the impetus for developing our thinking about MBT–C. In particular, our ideas about working in a time-limited manner were influenced by the Norwegian work on time-limited developmental therapy (e.g., Gydal & Knudtzon, 2002; Haugvik & Johns, 2006, 2008; Johns, 2008; Svendsen, Tanum Johns, Brautaset, & Egebjerg, 2012). At the same time, we have been influenced by the sea change that has taken place in the attitude to working with parents; no longer seen as simply an adjunct to the child's therapy, parent work has rightly come to be seen as central to therapeutic change. As the title of Novick and Novick's (2005) seminal book puts it, "Working with parents makes therapy work." So when the American Psychological Association offered us an opportunity to write a book about MBT with children, five members of the original working group came together, drawing on our experience in a number of clinical settings and in close collaboration with each of our clinical teams, to develop and describe a model of time-limited MBT–C in a form that we hope can speak to child therapists from a range of clinical and conceptual backgrounds and that is applicable to work in a variety of settings with diverse children and parents.

The work described in this book thus draws its inspiration from a number of settings and contexts, in clinics across the United Kingdom, Europe, and North America. Nicole Muller is a child and family psychotherapist based at the De Jutters Centre for Child and Youth Mental Health in The Hague, Netherlands, where she and her team have extensive experience offering time-limited MBT to children and families with attachment disorders, trauma, or emerging personality disorder. As well as running introductory and advanced MBT–C trainings, Muller has written several articles about MBT for children and families and has a particular interest in work with fostered and adopted children (Muller, 2011; Muller, Gerits, & Siecker, 2012). Both Norka Malberg and Nick Midgley trained as psychodynamic child psychotherapists and worked at the Anna Freud Centre in London; they have been members of the clinical team there that developed a model of MBT for families (MBT–F; Asen & Fonagy, 2012a, 2012b; Keaveny et al., 2012). Nick Midgley has continued to develop this work with a particular focus on MBT for looked-after and adopted children (Midgley et al., 2017), including a mentalization-based model of psychoeducation, the Reflective Fostering Programme. After moving to the United States, Norka Malberg continued to develop her thinking about MBT with children in private practice, as well as during her 2-year tenure as clinical director of the Home Visiting Early Intervention Project in Connecticut. One of her particular areas of interest is in working with parents in the child therapy context (Malberg, 2015). Karin Ensink, now a professor of child and adolescent psychology at Université Laval in Québec, Canada, also worked as a clinician and researcher at the Anna Freud Centre and did her doctorate work on the development of children's mentalizing capacities with Peter Fonagy and Mary Target. Her focus is on mentalization, trauma, and psychopathology in children, adolescents, and parents. As part of her work in Québec, she has contributed to elaborating a model of MBT for children and parents with histories of trauma and personality difficulties (Ensink & Normandin, 2011). Karin Lindqvist is a clinical psychologist working with children and adolescents in foster care, as well as their parents and foster parents. She also holds a part-time research assistant position at the Erica Foundation in Stockholm, Sweden, where she trained in mentalization-based work with children and parents. The Erica Foundation offers professional training at the university level and also psychodynamic and mentalization-based mental health services to children, adolescents, and families; it developed one of the first intensive trainings for child psychotherapists seeking to use an MBT approach with children. The Erica Foundation has been a pioneer in evaluating the effectiveness of a short-term psychodynamic–MBT model for children and adolescents (Thorén, Pertoft Nemirovski, & Lindqvist, 2016).

As our backgrounds indicate, we share interest and training in psychodynamic therapy with children and have all been influenced by the development of MBT that has taken place at the Anna Freud Centre in London, as well as elsewhere in the United States and Europe. However, the contexts in which we have developed our ideas have been somewhat different, and the approach described in this book tries to provide a synthesis of what we (and the teams that we have each been a part of) have learned. In presenting this shared model, we acknowledge the vital input we have received from colleagues working on each of our teams in developing and describing this approach to time-limited MBT–C.

What should be made clear, however, is that the specific model described in this book has not yet been subjected to systematic evaluation, beyond an initial naturalistic outcome study at the Erica Foundation (Thorén, Pertoft Nemirovski, & Lindqvist, 2016), and as such it remains a clinical guide for an approach to treatment that is not yet evidence based. Many of the components of the model are explicitly rooted in empirical findings, and as mentioned earlier, MBTs have shown themselves to be effective with different clinical populations, including adults with BPD (Bateman & Fonagy, 2009), adolescents who self-harm (Rossouw & Fonagy, 2012), and parents and at-risk infants (Slade, Sadler, et al., 2005). The particular model of MBT set out in this book, however, with its focus on time-limited work for children in middle childhood, will need to be systematically evaluated before we can say with more certainty what works, for whom, under what circumstances, and in what conditions.

AN OUTLINE OF THIS BOOK

This book is divided into two parts—the first primarily theoretical, the second mostly clinical. Readers who are already familiar with the concept of mentalization and the empirical and developmental research around it may wish to skip the first part; but even for those whose interest is purely clinical, we would encourage you to engage with the theoretical section first. After all, MBT is based on the idea that learning a set of behaviors (e.g., mentalization-promoting therapeutic techniques) is not sufficient in itself;

what is important is the intentions that inform those behaviors—intentions that ultimately depend on a way of thinking about the world, in other words, theory. For this reason, the first chapter provides an overview of the concept of mentalizing, specifically focusing on mentalization in children and what we might expect to see during middle childhood. In the second chapter, we describe the situations in which a child's mentalizing might be underdeveloped or how to recognize when mentalizing has broken down. We offer some provisional thoughts on the links between these mentalizing difficulties and the kind of clinical problems that often bring children and families to seek help. These first two chapters are intended to offer a conceptual background for the model of time-limited MBT–C that is described in the remaining parts of the book.

The second part of the book begins with a general introduction to time-limited MBT–C, setting out the basic model and the framework, then outlining who may be suitable for this way of working. Because we consider the mentalizing stance a foundation for all the clinical work in MBT–C, whether in working with children or their parents, this is the focus of Chapter 4 and is deliberately presented before we go into details about MBT techniques. Chapter 5 describes the process of assessment of children in MBT–C, discussing aspects that are especially relevant to assessment from a mentalizing perspective as well as the practicalities of the assessment of both child and parents. We then go on to describe the therapeutic interventions used in the direct work with children in Chapter 6, followed by a description of clinical work with parents from an MBT–C perspective in Chapter 7. Following a chapter on working toward ending treatment, the book ends with a case study that provides an example of what a complete case might look like in time-limited MBT–C, followed by some reflections on potential future developments and final thoughts on future developments for MBT–C. The Appendix lists some of the measures that clinicians can use to assess reflective functioning in children and their parents.

This book is a guide for clinicians rather than a full treatment manual and is intended to be used flexibly, according to the setting and contexts in which the reader may work. Throughout the book, we make use of clinical vignettes, which we hope will help the reader gain a sense of how the MBT–C model looks in practice. These vignettes are based on composite cases, which draw on our clinical experience but do not describe actual children or families. Although such fictionalized cases always face the risk that the work can be presented in an idealized form and that the messy reality of clinical practice can be airbrushed out, we have made an effort not to present these as examples of "perfect" therapy but to portray usual clinical practice, with all its imperfections and improvisation.

I

THEORETICAL FRAMEWORK

1

THE DEVELOPMENT OF MENTALIZING

Mentalization refers to the uniquely human ability to interpret the meaning of others' behavior by considering their underlying mental states and intentions, as well as the capacity to understand the impact of one's own affects and behaviors on others (Fonagy & Target, 1996b; 2000; Target & Fonagy, 1996). In simpler language, mentalizing is about understanding oneself and others on the basis of what's going on inside us; it involves *keeping mind in mind* and *seeing oneself from the outside and others from the inside*. If that sounds rather cognitive, then Allen and Fonagy (2006) helpfully reminds us that, at its most meaningful, mentalizing is "suffused with emotion" (p. 8). Indeed, when we are mentalizing well, we are likely to be able to

- have an awareness of what we are feeling as well as a sense of our personalities or qualities as people, which helps us have a sense of how we "look from the outside" to others, so that it is in turn easier to understand their reactions to us;

http://dx.doi.org/10.1037/0000028-002
Mentalization-Based Treatment for Children: A Time-Limited Approach, by N. Midgley, K. Ensink, K. Lindqvist, N. Malberg, and N. Muller

- have a solid ability to consider the emotions and motivations of others, and see their reactions and behaviors from this perspective;
- have some awareness of the limits of our ability to know what is in the minds of others;
- show some curiosity about how the world looks from other people's perspectives and how our own perspective may influence what we do or color how we see someone else's behavior; and
- be mindful that we might get it wrong when we try to understand why others behave in the way they do and that trying to make sense of these misunderstandings can enrich our interpersonal relationships.

This chapter provides an introduction to the concept of mentalizing and draws on developmental research to demonstrate how the capacity to mentalize emerges across the course of childhood and early adolescence. It outlines the development in understanding of self and others as *intentional mental agents* and uses empirical research to show the importance of this to emotional well-being and mental health. Because this book focuses on middle childhood (roughly between the ages of 5 and 12), we try to set out the particular features of mentalizing at this stage of life and attempt to answer some common questions that clinicians may have about mentalization. In doing so, we hope this chapter will provide a conceptual foundation for the model of time-limited mentalization-based treatment for children (MBT–C) that is set out in the later chapters of this book.

WHY MENTALIZING MATTERS

Tom (age 9) is a kind-hearted, helpful, and generous boy who is generally well-liked and who has a number of close friends. His teachers complain that he frequently does not finish his work because he is distracted and prefers to chat and socialize. This also causes trouble at home because he relies on his father to bail him out. He will often say that he has done all his work, and at the last minute, just before going to bed, his parents will discover that half his work has not been done. He also frequently forgets things, either at school or at home.

One morning, Tom and his father are about to arrive at school when Tom suddenly realizes that he left his lunchbox on the kitchen table. They turn around and head back home in the morning traffic. Realizing that he will be late for a meeting at work, Tom's father spends the next 15 minutes berating Tom for his lack of organization and goes through the list of Tom's shortcomings. As they arrive home, Tom's mother opens the door to hand the lunchbox to a tearful and angry Tom, who says, "It's not fair; Dad's been shouting at me all the way home." Both mother and son knows Tom's father can be intimidating when angry, so Mom shoots Tom a glance that Tom thinks is telling him, "You'll be OK; you can handle it." She says, "Your dad may be overreacting, but he's worried about being late for his meeting— let's talk tonight."

When Tom gets back in the car, he feels a bit less upset and tells his father he is sorry but to please stop shouting at him. Tom knows that his father loves him and spends hours helping him with projects and homework; he understands that this helps him to earn good grades. Being able to access these positive images of his father helps him recover quickly and not dwell too long on the hurtful comments his father made. From past experience, he knows that when his father is angry, he says things he doesn't mean. He also knows something about his father's personality, partly because he has heard his mother and father discuss this, and his father saying that he regrets shouting. Tom's dad usually appreciates it when his wife intervenes when he goes "over the limit" because he knows it is difficult for everyone. Tom likes it when his mom is playful and funny and when she diffuses their arguments by saying to his father, in a matter-of-fact and joking way, "Well, I would never have thought of Tom as immature; I think it's just a case of ordinary, garden-variety laziness that we all know too well," making his father laugh.

Tom's increasing awareness of how others are likely to view his behavior is a double-edged sword, and although this gives him an advantage in playing the social game, it also makes him more concerned about what others think. For example, he knows not to retaliate when a classmate with Asperger syndrome punches him when he accidentally bumps into him. But Tom still doesn't understand why this boy doesn't receive the same punishment he would have received for the same act. However, he's becoming increasingly interested in understanding why people behave the way they do. Although he pretends to be playing computer games, he listens intently when his parents talk to each other or his aunts about what is happening in the family and the various personal and relationship challenges his older cousins are facing.

In this example, it is clear that by age 9, Tom knows what he feels, is able to articulate this, and has already built a rich understanding of his parents' personalities; he is developing an increasingly sophisticated repertoire of explanations for why people behave the way they do. He is also coming to understand himself, his personality, and his own strengths and weaknesses. Sometimes he can use this to help better manage his own behavior. In addition to knowing more generally that when people get angry, they sometimes say things they don't mean, his understanding of his father helps him not to be unduly phased by his father's anger. These feelings are balanced by a secure knowledge of his father's love and an appreciation for his care and help. Furthermore, Tom's knowledge of himself makes it easy for him to brush off his father's comments about him being immature. All of this may look and sound quite straightforward—and for most of us, most of the time, it is. But what Tom is demonstrating here is a capacity to mentalize, including an ability to take the other's perspective and to use his own understanding of why people behave the way they do to manage his own emotional responses.

In this example, we can see that this mentalization capacity underpins a developing sense of self: Tom no longer depends on his mother to explain why his father gets angry, and his sense of himself does not change when his father calls him immature because he has a sense of who he is and that his father is probably just saying this because he is angry. We see how, as Fonagy, Gergely, Jurist, and Target (2002) put it, mentalization is central to the sense of self and affect regulation. Being able to mentalize, even in a fairly stressful situation as when his dad is angry with him, helps Tom to stay emotionally regulated. It helps him make sense of the situation, so he can see it in perspective and remain focused on the priorities. Allen and Fonagy (2006) described this function of mentalizing as like having a pause button, which can be used to help regulate our emotional reactions. Given that Tom has a secure relationship with his father and gets a great deal of help from seeing his mother explain his father's behavior, it is clear that this protects Tom from feeling that he is bad inside. So even when being criticized by his father, Tom's self-worth doesn't collapse, and he is better able to accept his need to change. Tom probably stands to gain more than he would lose from this opportunity to learn about anger and aggression, and he will not be intimidated when he encounters aggression in peers or later in life. Here we see how important mentalization is, especially in close relationships, and how it can transform even difficult experiences. As Fonagy and Allison (2014) noted, the stakes are highest in close interpersonal relationships, especially attachment relationships in which general emotional understanding is not enough and a more nuanced understanding of others, as well as of our own feelings and personalities and the impact of this on others, can have important implications for the quality of these relationships.

When we are able to make sense of the behaviors of others (and ourselves), the interpersonal world becomes a more predictable, safe, and meaningful place. But when we misread the intentions of others, or struggle to make sense of our own internal states, this can lead to confusion, misunderstanding, and difficulties in interpersonal relating, contributing to escalating conflict or bottled up anger and fear. How we interpret why people are behaving in the way they do has a huge impact on the way we think and behave.

Quite often, children and parents are not familiar with the word *mentalizing*, and children ask whether it means the same as *mental*—in the context of being mad or "crazy." Parents often ask whether the term means the same as mindfulness, empathy, or emotional understanding. Those who are familiar with developmental research literature may ask us how the concept relates to terms such as *theory of mind, mind-mindedness,* or even *social cognition.*

The term *mentalization* has its roots in 1960s French psychoanalytic terminology (Marty, 1991), but the modern use of the term owes much to the work of Peter Fonagy, Antony Bateman, Mary Target, and their colleagues, who since the 1990s have made a unique contribution in pulling together diverse lines of inquiry and bridging the divides across disciplines to develop an integrated, developmentally based model of mentalization. This emerged out of work on understanding the process of change in child psychoanalysis (Fonagy & Target, 1998) and developments in the treatment of adults with borderline personality disorder (Bateman & Fonagy, 2004). Although we agree that the term is not always easy to explain to children and families, the oddness of the word can be helpful as a way of "marking" this capacity as something that we try to focus on in an MBT.

Mentalizing can be thought of as an umbrella concept (Luyten & Fonagy, 2015; Sharp, 2006) that overlaps and encompasses a number of other important constructs. *Theory of mind* (Premack & Woodruff, 1978), for example, overlaps with some of the more cognitive elements of mentalizing, whereas *empathy* tends to focus more on the emotional aspect of perspective-taking and is mostly used in relation to others. The concepts of *mindfulness* and mentalizing are often compared (Masterpasqua, 2016) and certainly share a recognition of the importance of taking a curious, open, and accepting attitude toward mental states. (For those interested in this topic, there are excellent discussions of the relationships between all these terms and more in Choi-Kain & Gunderson, 2008, and Kim, 2015.)

Because the term *reflective functioning* is used later in this book, it is worth saying a bit more about this concept here. The terms *mentalization* and *reflective function* are often used interchangeably, although reflective function was initially considered to refer to the measurement of mentalization as manifested within narratives regarding attachment relationships. In this book, we use reflective functioning to refer to the capacity to mentalize, especially explicit mentalizing, that is, the conscious ability to stop and reflect on the states of mind of self and other.

Just as mentalizing overlaps with other terms, the concept also contains within it a number of dimensions that can be helpful to disentangle when working clinically. Although our colleagues have identified several of these (Luyten, Fonagy, Lowyck, & Vermote, 2012), there are two that we have found especially helpful when thinking about our work with children: the difference between explicit (or controlled) and implicit (or automatic) mentalizing and the difference between the mentalizing of self and other.

First, mentalization has both *implicit/automatic* and *explicit/controlled* dimensions. Most of the time, mentalization goes on automatically, without us needing to put things into words. Without consciously thinking about it, we infer people's mental states, often based on their expressions in the eye regions of the face and feel that we know when they seem to be angry, happy, sad, frightened, interested, or bored. From an evolutionary perspective, rapid processing of social information was essential in identifying whether others were potential friends who we could cooperate with to increase the chances of success in complex tasks and survival or potential foes who were a threat to our security. Speed of processing is of essence where detection of threat is concerned because it is a matter of life and death, but this automatic processing has the disadvantage of being based on, and therefore biased by previous experience. It is not adapted for more complex social situations in which slower consideration and figuring out possible motives are necessary to make accurate inferences. In the earlier example, when Tom's mother glanced at him as he arrived home, he could implicitly understand that she was intending to let him know that he'd be OK and that he could handle the situation. These nonverbal signals, like eye contact, turn-taking, and contingent responses, are mostly processed outside conscious awareness. Neuroscience researchers have studied this kind of *automatic, implicit mentalizing* and found that it seems to be subserved by a set of brain circuits that rely primarily on sensory information and that, from an evolutionary perspective, are quite primitive (Luyten & Fonagy, 2015). These include the amygdala, basal ganglia, and the dorsal anterior cingulate cortex, all of which are primarily involved in rapid detection of threats and social information related to the fight-or-flight response.

Although our implicit or automatic mentalizing may be quick and agile, it may not always be accurate. Considering that automatic mentalizing is largely based on prior experience, when past experiences have been overwhelmingly negative, this processing tends to be negatively biased. In these cases, past experience suggests that a high level of vigilance toward potential threat is needed and that it is potentially dangerous to trust others. However, this is unlikely to be appropriate in social contexts of low threat. There are times when children may feel suspicious and have a sense, for example, that someone might be trying to trick them and will need to stop and consider whether that judgment is correct. In other words, there are times when we may need to make use of more *explicit mentalizing*, a process that requires more conscious and explicit reflection on the emotions, thoughts, and intentions of others. Interestingly, neuroscientists suggest that this capacity is subserved by newer brain circuits, which are more linked with symbolic and linguistic processing, such as the lateral prefrontal cortex and the medial prefrontal cortex (Luyten & Fonagy, 2015). These are parts of the brain that are commonly activated by tasks involving reasoning, effortful control, and perspective-taking. Such processes may be slower than the more automatic modes of mentalizing, but they make it possible for us to more carefully and deliberately make attributions about the emotions, thoughts, and feelings of self and others. This allows us to consider whether our immediate reactions are actually warranted after we have considered the situation, and then we can override or adjust our first impressions to be in line with these reflections.

We often make use of more controlled or explicit mentalizing when there has been a difficult situation that demands some kind of active reflection to help make sense of it. For example, in the vignette described earlier in the chapter, Tom's mother has to think carefully about how to intervene in a way that would diffuse the situation and signal to Tom's father that he needs to step back and cool down. She tried to do this in a way that limited the chances he would feel undermined, while protecting Tom and monitoring whether he was becoming fearful and dysregulated. At the same time, the situation challenged Tom's father, who at times can be highly reflective, generous, and empathic, to regain his mentalizing capacity. When he loses this capacity, he is more likely to misread his son's agitation as intentional and willful opposition, rather than triggered in part by his own anger.

The examples given so far largely focus on the capacity to mentalize others, but mentalizing also takes place in relation to the self. For example, Tom's father may reflect on his temper and the impact this has on his family; he may actively think of ways he can maintain self-awareness and mentally step back when he becomes too frustrated and disengage so that he can regain control. On this basis, he may decide not to take Tom to school on mornings when he has early meetings at work. The capacity to explicitly mentalize about one's own thoughts and feelings is thus an essential part of managing relationships and modulating one's own emotional responses. Furthermore, Tom's increasing understanding of himself and awareness of some of his weaknesses helps him to develop strategies to balance his desire to be liked and to work on his "air-headedness." Similarly, children and adults who can quickly lose their tempers, as Tom's father does, have to work at being conscious of the impact of this trait on others.

Although it does not distinguish among the different components described earlier, for children in middle childhood, clinical researchers, including the authors of this book, have developed a way of assessing a child's capacity for reflective functioning, using the Child and Adolescent Reflective Functioning Scale (CRFS; Ensink, Normandin, et al., 2015; Ensink, Target, Oandasan, & Duval, 2015). The CRFS is used to code the Child Attachment Interview (CAI; Target, Fonagy, Shmueli-Goetz, Schneider, & Datta, 2000), a semistructured interview in which children (aged 7–12) are asked to describe themselves and their relationships with their parents. Table 1.1 shows the different codings (−1 to 9) that may be used to try and assess a child's reflective

TABLE 1.1
Different Levels of Child Reflective Functioning

Level	Description
−1	Bizarre, disorganized response in which mentalizing is actively avoided or there is an aggressive refusal to mentalize: *When Mom gets cross? There is an angel dancing on her shoe.*
0	Absence of mentalization: *I don't know, it just is.*
1	Descriptions in terms of physical or behavioral nonmental characteristics: *Mom says, "Go to your room."*
3	Unelaborated references to mental states when describing relationships: *I like it. It's fun.*
4	References to mental states but with gaps that have to be filled in: *When I feel sad, my mom like . . . comforts me.*
5	Clear description showing a solid mental-state understanding, even if fairly simple: *When Mom gets angry, she shouts, and I don't like it, but I know she doesn't really mean what she says and that I am a little bit to blame.*
7–9	Increasingly sophisticated mental-state understanding, with 9 denoting exceptional mental-state understanding: *When Dad gets angry, I also get angry at first, but then I feel guilty, because I know he helps me a lot. And when I forget my books at school, trying to finish my homework takes much longer, and he gets tired and has work to do, too.*

Note. From "Maternal and Child Reflective Functioning in the Context of Child Sexual Abuse: Pathways to Depression and Externalising Difficulties," by K. Ensink, M. Bégin, L. Normandin, and P. Fonagy, 2016, *European Journal of Psychotraumatology, 7*, p. 4. Copyright 2016 by Karin Ensink, Michaël Bégin, Lina Normandin, and Peter Fonagy. Adapted with permission.

capacity, with examples of the kind of things a child might say that would lead to that coding.

Thinking about these codings from a clinical perspective, some broad pointers may be useful. First, when a child responds in a bizarre and disorganized way, or where there appears to be an active avoidance of mentalization or an aggressive refusal to mentalize, this is a particular cause for concern. The therapist should try and develop an understanding of what underlies these responses and whether they can be adequately explained by cognitive immaturity or are triggered by anxiety in response to the invitation to reflect and express their thoughts. Sometimes the child becomes silly or angry when invited to mentalize, or the response may be related to the child becoming disorganized. When there are many of these types of responses, the therapist should carefully monitor whether the child continues to manifest these types of responses or whether they increase in the context of the therapy or rapidly decrease as the child begins to feel more secure with the therapist.

When children show no evidence of mentalizing (Level 0) or only think about themselves and others in physical and behavioral terms (Level 1), this is obviously a cause for concern. As a broad guideline, we ideally hope to see school-age children show a basic understanding of themselves, others, and relationships in mental state terms (rating Level 4 or 5). If a child shows some capacity to identify feelings or mental states (Level 3), this is an indication that he or she could benefit from additional help in elaborating a more solid, even if incomplete, mental understanding of self, others, and relationships. When a child appears to be functioning below a Level 3, this could be a cause of concern in terms of them being able to use basic mentalizing to deal with the challenges of life.

FACTORS THAT PROMOTE THE CAPACITY TO MENTALIZE

Although the capacity to mentalize is partly an innate one in humans with its own biological underpinnings (Kovács, Teglas, & Endress, 2010), there is little doubt that the development of our ability to mentalize also depends on the quality of the social learning environment in which we are raised. In their major work, *Affect Regulation, Mentalization and the Development of the Self*, Fonagy et al. (2002) proposed a developmental model in which awareness of mental states emerges in the context of early attachment relationships. They showed how children learn to identify and mentally represent their own affects through the parents' interest in the child's subjective experience and the parents' emotional displays focusing on the child's mind and feelings. In this model, the parents' capacity to imagine the subjective experience of their infant or young child is considered to facilitate the development of affect regulation and self-control. They may do this through attention-shifting strategies to regulate distress. For example, a parent may direct his or her child's attention to the picture of a cute dog on the wall to help shift attention away from a nurse who is about to give the child an injection. Or after the injection, a parent may help by offering a representation of and communication about affects (e.g., "I could see you trying to be brave, even though it hurt a little when the nurse did that. But then it was over and not as bad as you had thought it would be. Wow, you handled that well!"). Such mind-minded communications gradually help children start thinking of themselves as people with a mind, able to use words and thoughts in a way that allows a shift toward self-regulation and self-control (Fonagy et al., 2002).

The Importance of Reflective Parenting and the Pedagogical Stance

As the seminal work of John Bowlby and his colleagues has shown, the quality of early caregiving relationships is crucial for children's social and emotional development, given that infants are totally dependent on their caregivers for all their basic needs for survival, security, and protection.

Because infants are born without their own capacity to reestablish emotional regulation when faced with distress, they rely on their caregivers to help them regulate when they are frightened or overwhelmed. Through this process of dyadic regulation, in which parents repeatedly help the infants to reestablish self-regulation, children gradually learn to regulate themselves (Trevarthen, Aitken, Vandekerckove, Delafield-Butt, & Nagy, 2006).

Because they are unable to articulate their feelings and distress, infants and young children depend on the parent's interest in their subjective experience, and their capacity to make the child's behavior meaningful by interpreting it in terms of underlying mental states. Reflective functioning is seen as underlying sensitive responding by helping parents to mentally put themselves in the place of the infant and imagine the infant's experience (Fonagy & Target, 1997). From this perspective, *reflective parenting* (Cooper & Redfern, 2016) can be seen as an orientation in which the child's mind is kept in mind (Slade, 2005); a *reflective parenting stance* is implicit in interactions (Ensink, Bégin, Normandin, & Fonagy, 2016) and might include the following features:

- a benign interest in the mind of the child and emotional availability to help the child make sense of his or her own reactions and those of others;
- a capacity to look past the child's behavior to determine what it communicates about his or her experience, feelings, and difficulties;
- a capacity to play, joke, and imagine with the child;
- a motivation to consider the meaning and sense of a child's thoughts and feelings, even if one cannot be exactly sure what is in the child's mind;
- availability to help the child put feelings into words and elaborate autobiographically meaningful narratives;
- a motivation to see the child's perspective and awareness that the child's experience may be very different from one's own;
- an ability to have a sense of one's own thoughts and feelings when interacting with the child and modulate one's own aggression; and/or
- an appreciation that one's own feelings and moods will affect, and have an impact on, one's children.

As with children, clinical researchers have developed a way of assessing reflective functioning in parents by using a Reflective Functioning Scale, which is used to code the Parent Development Interview (PDI; Slade, Aber, Bresgi, Berger, & Kaplan, 2004). Using this scale, Slade and her colleagues have been able to code the way parents speak about their relationship with their children to assess explicit parental reflective functioning. Table 1.2 shows the different ratings that can be given (-1 to 9) and gives examples of the way a parent might speak that would lead to a given rating. Although the PDI is not a clinical tool, it can be helpful for clinicians to have this system of coding in mind when thinking about what good (or poor) mentalizing may look like in the way parents speak about their relationship to their child. Recently, a way of assessing reflective parenting implicit in interaction with young children has also been developed and can be used conjointly with the PDI to identify strengths and difficulties in parents mentalizing (Ensink, Leroux, Normandin, Biberdzic, & Fonagy, in press).

TABLE 1.2
Different Levels of Parental Reflective Functioning

Level	Description
−1	Bizarre, disorganized response in which mentalizing is actively avoided or there is an aggressive refusal to mentalize: Parent: *When I am talking on the phone with friends, she provokes me by running up and down, and the only thing that helps to calm her is to hit her.*
0	Absence of mentalization: Parent: *He just does it for no reason; he's just like that.*
1	Descriptions in terms of physical or behavioral nonmental characteristics: Parent: *He just keeps twirling around—he never stops.*
3	Unelaborated references to mental states when describing relationships: Parent: *He gets irritable.*
4	References to mental states but with gaps that have to be filled in: Parent: *When we are preparing for an exam and he messes around, I know it is going to take so much longer. I get so angry.*
5	Clear description showing a solid mental-state understanding, even if fairly simple: Parent: *I get angry because he loses everything—his gloves, his books— and when we arrived at school, and he had forgotten his gloves again and we had to turn back, I realized I was going to be late for work, and I lost it. But I realize that I need to find a way to help him become more responsible, and it doesn't help to shout.*
7–9	Increasingly sophisticated mental-state understanding, with 9 denoting exceptional and complete mental-state understanding: Parent: *I don't often get angry with him, but sometimes when he becomes very excited and maybe because he wants to show off in front of his friends, he behaves in a way that he would not usually, becoming defiant, and I feel a little foolish and frustrated. He does not realize that he actually risks losing his friends' respect, and it makes them feel uncomfortable. I don't know how to explain this without hurting his feelings.*

Note. From "Maternal and Child Reflective Functioning in the Context of Child Sexual Abuse: Pathways to Depression and Externalising Difficulties," by K. Ensink, M. Bégin, L. Normandin, and P. Fonagy, 2016, *European Journal of Psychotraumatology, 7*, p. 4. Copyright 2016 by Karin Ensink, Michaël Bégin, Lina Normandin, and Peter Fonagy. Adapted with permission.

Fonagy, Steele, Steele, Moran, and Higgitt (1991) proposed that the parent's mentalizing stance has implications for infant attachment because mentalizing underlies sensitive parenting. Consistent with this, there is evidence that parents' reflective functioning about their attachment relationships, both past and present, underlies sensitivity in interaction with infants and that higher reflective functioning is associated with fewer negative behaviors (Ensink, Normandin, Plamondon, Berthelot, & Fonagy, 2016; Slade, Grienenberger, Bernbach, Levy, & Locker, 2005; Suchman, DeCoste, Leigh, & Borelli, 2010). In an important study of intergenerational patterns of attachment, Fonagy, Steele, Steele, Higgitt, and Target (1994) were able to show how mothers with a history of deprivation who are able to acquire a capacity for reflective functioning are more likely to have infants with a secure attachment. The value of mindful or reflective parenting in the development of affect regulation and secure attachment in the child has been demonstrated in a number of empirical studies (e.g., Ensink, Bégin, Normandin, & Fonagy, 2016; Koren-Karie, Oppenheim, Dolev, Sher, & Etzion-Carasso, 2002; Meins, Fernyhough, Fradley, & Tucker, 2001; Slade, Grienenberger, Bernbach, Levy, & Locker, 2005). For example mothers' reflective functioning about their own early attachment relationships has been shown to be associated with secure and organized infant attachment (Ensink, Normandin, Plamondon, Berthelot, & Fonagy, 2016), and associated with less externalizing difficulties in children (Ensink, Bégin, Normandin, & Fonagy, 2016). In fact, evidence from one study suggests that in the context of child sexual abuse, which disrupts affect regulation and triggers children's needs for security, maternal reflective functioning may have a particularly important role because it appears to counterbalance the effect of abuse (Ensink, Bégin, Normandin, Biberdzic, Vohl, & Fonagy, 2016). In the context of taking care of infants, reflective functioning is thought to promote sensitive parenting by helping parents look beyond behaviors to what the child is feeling and inhibit negative interactions by helping parents regulate their own negative reactions and remain focused on the child's needs. Even when their baby is distressed, these parents are able (at least most of the time) to remain relatively calm and not take it personally when their infant is dysregulated. This in turn helps the infant to become regulated (Ensink, Bégin, Normandin, & Fonagy, 2016). These patterns of feeling secure in the belief that others will be there when in distress or alternatively, trying to rely on the self to regulate, have been shown to have long-term implications for the way individuals regulate distress. It also underlies the feeling that it is safe and rewarding to express and share feelings with others when distressed, and in turn be available and supportive of others when they are in distress (Ensink, Bégin, Normandin, & Fonagy, 2016).

Secure attachment relationships provide optimal conditions for the development of mentalization, and not surprisingly, children and adults who are secure with regard to attachment also tend to see themselves and their significant relationships in terms of mental states more than others with insecure attachment styles. Furthermore, parental reflective functioning has been shown to remain important for school-age children's psychological adjustment (Ensink, Bégin, Normandin, & Fonagy, 2016) and to be a protective factor in the context of trauma. It is also associated with the development of reflective functioning in children (Ensink, Normandin, et al., 2015) and adolescents (Benbassat & Priel, 2012). In sum, the family is the key context in which children develop their capacity to mentalize, especially in relation to negative or distressing situations. One could say that one of the most important tasks of parents is to transmit a mentalizing stance and help their children become aware of their feelings and behaviors and use mentalizing to enhance and deepen their close relationships.

Natural Pedagogy and the Early Roots of Mentalizing, the Self, and Epistemic Trust

One of the questions that has intrigued both developmental researchers and clinicians is the ways in which parents communicate an interest in infants' mind and feelings and thereby help them to develop their own capacity to recognize and know their feelings and regulate emotions. From infancy onward, children are progressively building a type of autobiographical narrative of self in relation to others that is presymbolic, procedural, and involves nonverbal memories of sensory and affective experiences (Beebe & Stern, 1977; Fonagy & Target, 1996b). But what is the mechanism through which this development takes place?

Fonagy and colleagues (2002) drew on the work of Csibra and Gergely (2009) to propose that there are a set of recognizable ways through which caregivers transmit knowledge about the way relationships work to their offspring, referred to as *natural pedagogy*, referring to the various means that we as humans have—in a way that is quite specific to our species—for engaging in a quite extraordinarily rapid process of social teaching and learning. But how do babies know what information is important for them, and how do parents manage to signal to their infants that what they are communicating is of importance? Csibra and Gergely suggested that we do this through a series of *ostensive cues*, which for parents of babies might include things such as eye contract, turn-taking, and a special vocal tone ("mother-ese"), all of which help the infant to preferentially attend to what is being communicated. In more recent work, Fonagy and Allison (2014) suggested that these cues also serve to moderate what they called *natural epistemic vigilance*, that is, "the self-protective suspicion toward information coming from others that may be potentially damaging, deceptive or inaccurate" (p. 373). In other words, certain ways of verbal and nonverbal communicating (and building on this, certain relationships) not only communicate to infants that this information is of value but also that the person communicating with them is someone who is trustworthy—someone they can learn from.

Although the names used for these processes may seem confusing to some, we think these concepts are valuable not only for developmental researchers but also for clinicians, as we try to demonstrate in later chapters. In particular, we find it helpful to understand how parents' *contingent and congruent marked affect mirroring* is central in the early development of recognition of self and affective states and self-regulation. By this, Fonagy and Allison (2014) mean the way that, in emotionally charged interactions with their infant

- parents *partially* reflect the infant's affect, but at a lower level of intensity;
- in a way that fairly accurately reflects the infant's state of mind (congruent);
- in a timely manner, after the infant's affective display (contingent); and
- mark it, for example, with an exaggerated facial display or vocalization to signal to the infant that they recognize the feeling (e.g., fear or distress) but aren't experiencing it themselves in the same way.

The "marked" nature of this mirroring, which may have something of a play-acting quality, is especially important. By this, Fonagy et al. (2002) were referring to the exaggerated facial expressions and vocalizations that parents intuitively use when interacting with infants that makes it clear that they are trying to describe what the infant is feeling but in a way that also communicates that it is the child's own feelings that are being shown, not the adult's. For example, when a baby starts to cry, the caregiver may respond with an exaggerated facial reaction marked with a quizzical look and accompanied with calming words that name the infant's affect and possible mental states: "You look a little sad. Are you getting tired or feeling hungry? Don't worry, it won't be long." Insofar as the infant's feelings are being "marked," it is clear that it is not the caregiver who is feeling upset or hungry.

It is frequently said that infants find themselves in the loving gaze of the mother who sensitively picks up and mirrors the moment-to-moment changes in their affect states (Winnicott, 1967). By having their affects mirrored in this way, infants receive feedback that helps them develop basic representations of what their feelings look like, a building block for later being able to mentalize about oneself. Infants in turn appear exquisitely sensitive to this communication from the parent, as has been observed in microanalytic studies of mother–infant interaction (Beebe et al., 2012). Stern (2010) described this as a dance between parent and infant in which the rhythm and "feeling" of what it is like to relate is established. Some things that we take for granted, such as infants' need to be held, touched, and cuddled, may also play quite a central role in helping develop a sense of feeling comfortable and secure in one's body. In sum, the affective core of the self (Panksepp & Biven, 2012) can be seen as constellating around these early experiences of being held (Fonagy & Target, 2007a, 2007b). Furthermore, through these early experiences, the child develops an ongoing expectation of sensitive responding from others and of *epistemic trust*, that is, a "willingness to consider new knowledge from another person as trustworthy, generalizable and relevant to the self" (Fonagy & Allison, 2014, p. 373). Such expectations can help to reduce our natural epistemic vigilance, so that children can open themselves to learn from those around them and turn to them when in need. The establishment of epistemic trust can be seen as a precondition for the transmission of all knowledge that is culturally transmitted.

Through repeated experiences of marked affect mirroring, children learn to recognize their feelings, first how they look and then what they are called, contributing to an early sense of self. What starts as undifferentiated states of discomfort or tension become recognized as affects. At the same time, when parents mirror their infants' affect at a lower intensity, this is believed to help infants down-regulate their affect, until it is regulated. Insofar as infants experience themselves as initiating this interaction, they gain a sense of perceived control and agency (Fonagy, Gergely, & Target, 2007) and gradually become less reliant on the caregiver to help them regulate, until they are no longer dependent on dyadic regulation but have internalized a pattern of self-regulation.

The Role of Attention Control in the Establishment of Mentalizing

As one of the building blocks of mentalization, the concept of attention control is used in this book because we have found it to be helpful in clinical work with school-age children. The term was used by Fonagy and Target (2002), who argued that the development of self-regulation in infancy depends on the development of mechanisms to react to stress (affect regulation), maintain focused attention (regulation of attention), and interpret mental states in the self and others (explicit mentalizing). When operating in combination, these three mechanisms are "probably responsible for self-regulation in social relationships" (Fonagy & Target, 2002, p. 309), and their development is "arguably the most important evolutionary function of attachment to a caregiver" (p. 313). Although each can be thought of separately, in reality their functions are interdependent, with each feeding back to the others.

Affect regulation and explicit mentalizing are described elsewhere in this chapter, but it may be helpful to say a few words about the concept of attention control, which links directly to the ability to control impulsivity but also to function adequately in interpersonal contexts (Fonagy & Bateman, 2007). The word *attention* is used in a somewhat broader sense in this context than in the academic literature. Normally it is used to refer to the capacity to deliberately focus on some stimuli while deliberately excluding other types of information by controlling impulses to react to distracting stimuli. In the clinical literature about mentalization, attention regulation is described by Zevalkink, Verheugt-Pleiter, and Fonagy (2012) as the "ability to gain control of impulsiveness—something that can be learned in a safe relationship" (p. 145). During the first year of life, attention capacities are evident in the infant's capacity to orient and direct attention and later in "effortful control" (Beebe, Lachmann, & Jaffe, 1997), which makes a development leap during the second year of life. Parents frequently use distraction and redirection of attention to regulate their behavior and frustration. For example, if a mother says to a 2-year-old who is drawn to putting his fingers in electrical outlets, "Oh, you are angry because you cannot put your fingers in the plug," this mirroring of affect is likely to maintain the focus on exactly that which she does not want the child to do and increase his negative affect and frustration. It is more likely to be of value if the mother uses a process of defocusing from the undesirable object and refocusing the child's attention to something else, such as an interesting toy with which he can play, which will hopefully engage the child's interest and help him to disengage from the frustrating and dangerous situation but also reestablish emotion regulation. Later in childhood, as the child becomes increasingly self-regulating, attention control will take the form of a capacity to focus attention and to inhibit inappropriate responses. Furthermore, studies have suggested that the capacity to focus attention is associated with other abilities that develop in the context of secure attachment relationships, such as social competence, perspective-taking, and empathy (Fonagy & Target, 2002).

Parents can be viewed as organizers of attention systems (Fearon & Belsky, 2004), with the infant initially depending on the caregiver's regulatory capacity, or what has been called the "dyadic regulatory system" (Tronick, 2007). Kochanska, Coy, and Murray (2001) demonstrated how higher levels of mutual responsivity in mother–child dyads in the third year of life predict greater self-control and reduced need for maternal control. Attention regulation is seen as important in the development of the capacity to mentalize because "the ability to gain control of impulses that arise from within is an essential condition for the capacity to mentalize" (Zevalkink et al., 2012, p. 110).

THE CAPACITY TO MENTALIZE AT
DIFFERENT STAGES OF CHILDHOOD

MBT is a developmentally informed approach to therapy, and thus it is useful for clinicians to have some sense of the normal course of the development of emotional understanding and the sense of self in children across the early years because these are key dimensions of mentalization. By *normal*, we mean the capacities that children have usually achieved by different ages based on developmental studies, although of course there is great variation in when any particular child may do so. Nevertheless, if we consider what normally developing children are able to do from early on, it can help us to identify and appreciate the difficulties of the children and parents with whom we work, who may not have developed these basic abilities.

Children's understanding of mental states and emotions has been found to be consistently related to their present and future social competence (Eggum et al., 2011). For example, children with better emotion and mental state understanding are generally responded to more positively (Cassidy, Werner, Rourke, Zubernis, & Balaraman, 2003), are more likely to engage in positive play and cooperative pretend (Dunn & Brown, 1994), and use reasoning to try and resolve conflict (e.g., with siblings; Dunn, Slomkowski, Donelan, & Herrera, 1995) and to attempt reconciliation in the context of overt aggression (Liao, Li, & Su, 2014).

Emerging Understanding of Self, Others, and the Mind

Age 0 to 1 Year

During the first few months of life, infants are thought to begin to organize their experience and differentiate emotions by their valence (Widen & Russel, 2008), crystalizing around physical sensations of pleasure or pain and distress and how the parent responds to these. Infants appear to be biologically wired to be receptive to dyadic communication (Csibra & Gergely, 2009), attending to the parent's reactions and showing that they are sensitive to emotional communication. We know from microanalytic studies of mother–infant communication that infants are tuned in to the facial and physical reactions and tone of voice of the parent and react with disorientation and distress to inappropriate responding, such as when the parent laughs when the infant gets hurt or when the carer fails to respond to the infant's bids for communication (Beebe et al., 2012). By age 8 months, most infants are able to follow parents' gaze and engage in joint attention (Moore & Dunham, 1995; Tomasello & Farrar, 1986). This will become increasingly important in learning to focus attention and for both cognitive development and mutual and self-regulation strategies because it makes it possible to help infants self-regulate by distracting them from the source of distress and focus on something neutral or interesting. By 12 months, infants also show the ability to use the caregiver's reactions to know whether a new situation is safe and whether they can proceed and engage (Vaish, Grossmann, & Woodward, 2008)—for example, glancing at the mother to see whether she nods or shows a fearful face.

Age 1 to 3 Years

At around 15 to 18 months of age, a well-researched attachment milestone is reached, and distinct attachment patterns are evident in the way toddlers respond during separations and reunions in the context of the strange situation paradigm (Ainsworth, Blehar, Waters, & Wall, 1978). In this procedure developed to assess attachment, toddlers are observed during separations and reunions with their caregiver, and their responses are coded. Research using the strange situation has demonstrated that most toddlers have developed distinct patterns of regulating their distress based on repeated experiences of whether the mother was available and responded sensitively to their distress. These patterns form the well-known attachment strategies that have been validated across a range of cultures (van IJzendoorn & Kroonenberg, 1988). The experiment shows that toddlers have developed an internal model based on whether they can expect the parent to be available or unavailable to help them regulate distress or, alternatively, expect her to be frightening and increase distress.

At around 18 months, toddlers are also beginning to engage in pretend play and show an early capacity for self-awareness evident in their ability to recognize, when they look in the mirror, that the image in front of them is a reflection of themselves (Bukatko & Daehler, 2004)

During the toddler years, further rapid strides are made in self-regulation and mentalizing; at an individual level, cognitive and attentional processes mature, language skills emerge, and play with peers stimulates the development of a range of prosocial abilities. Fonagy and Target (1996b) theorized that between the ages of 2 and 3 years, play becomes an especially important realm where the child, entering a pretend mode, can discover the representational aspects of thoughts through the elaboration of different fantasy play scenarios. Especially when the parent is able to engage in playing and pretending with the child, this encourages both the process of imagining but also provides an opportunity for the child to see and learn something about how mental reality works.

Play is widely recognized to have an important developmental role in trying out roles, developing skills, and learning social abilities in humans as well as other mammals. Playing and suspending reality, while imagining and creating a realm of make belief, appears to be fertile ground for learning about mental states, developing affect regulation and empathy. Creating play narratives and finding different endings through play is thought to contribute to the sense that subjective experience can be expressed, transformed, and represented in different ways by the child (Slade, 1994). From a clinical perspective, children's fantasy play is an early mental activity that helps them integrate experience and make some sense of their own and others reactions, and thus facilitates self- and emotion regulation (Berk, Mann, & Ogan, 2006; McMahon, 2009).

From a neurocognitive perspective, play contributes to the development of higher cognitive functions and of the prefrontal regions implicated in inhibition and executive control underlying creative, self-reflective, and empathic capabilities (Panksepp, 2007). Consistent with this, brief play interventions have been shown to facilitate the development of a cognitive capacity referred to as executive function, and involved in self-control through attention and impulse regulation (Lillard et al., 2013).

Furthermore, we know from developmental research that children learn to think about mental states and the reflex to think in terms of them in the context of families where they have opportunities to learn and through relationships where they experience others as mentalizing and get help to develop these capacities themselves (Clarke-Stewart & Dunn, 2006; Denham & Kochanoff, 2002a, 2002b; Symons, Fossum, & Collins, 2006; Taumoepeau & Ruffman, 2008). Initially they may require active scaffolding by parents, but with practice most children internalize this as part of their own repertoire. Most likely without thinking about it consciously, reflective parents teach children to adopt a mentalizing stance themselves in the context of a range of everyday activities, for example, when a parent comments on the emotional reactions of a storybook character or uses conflict between siblings as a way to teach children to take each other's perspective. Furthermore, parents spontaneously engage in reminiscing about emotionally challenging and significant experiences and in this way help children to develop the capacity to elaborate a series of narratives around significant events that can be linked up into an autobiography.

With emerging language capacities opening doors to learning and exchanges about emotions, children's ability to express, understand, and communicate about feelings develops rapidly. By age 2 or 3 years, most children make reference to and recognize facial expressions of basic emotions such as happiness, sadness, fear, and anger in their everyday communication (Kring, 2008; Weimer, Sallquist, & Bolnick, 2012). During this period children go from an implicit knowledge of emotions to a conscious knowledge of them (Southam-Gerow & Kendall, 2002), and they also begin to use words such as *want*, *wish*, and *pretend*, reflecting the early use of language to express agency and self.

Age 3 to 4 Years

Children now start to show the ability to identify how others will feel in emotion-provoking situations. They know that others can want, like, dislike and feel, and how this is linked to how people will react. They can predict the reactions of others based on what they know about the likes and dislikes or desires and intentions of others (Denham et al., 2014). Children at this age usually show an awareness that the emotions of others can be different in the same situation, showing that they no longer egocentrically assume that others will feel the same way they do and suggesting that they can imagine the emotions of others, even before they are able to pass theory of mind tasks (discussed subsequently). For example, they know that although they will be happy to find a new toy, the child who lost it will be sad (Pons, Harris, & de Rosnay, 2004). From around age 3 years, words such as *thinking* and *knowing* also become part of the child's expressive vocabulary, showing an emerging implicit awareness of self as a mentalizing agent.

Age 4 to 5 Years

At this age, most children pass another well-researched milestone, the theory of mind or false-belief task (Happé & Frith, 2014; Premack & Woodruff, 1978). In this task, the child sees Maxi's mother moving the cookies from where they are usually kept in the blue cupboard to a green cupboard and has to predict where Maxi will look for the cookies. Correctly predicting that Maxi will have a false belief and look in the blue cupboard shows that the child has developed the *capacity to imagine and represent the mental perspective* of someone else. This demonstrates that children are no longer egocentric in their thinking, as are younger children who simply assume that others will think like they do and know what they know. At this age, some children who have specific difficulties (e.g., slightly more impulsive or aggressive temperaments) may develop an even better knowledge of emotion in this area if they have access to people who use situations where there are disagreements or conflict as opportunities to teach them about the impact of their behavior (Laurent & Ensink, 2016). This is thought to help them make interpersonal adjustments to compensate for their temperaments through other prosocial behavior so that they may not necessarily be less popular.

At this age, children also begin to be able to describe themselves, but this is still mainly in terms of physical characteristics and their likes and dislikes, for example, "I am a boy, I have blue eyes, and I love dogs and playing soccer." At this age, self-representations are often overly positive and infused with fantasies about what they want to be or qualities that they wish to have

(Trzesniewski, Kinal, & Donnellan, 2010), which may contrast with their actual feelings of vulnerability.

Age 5 to 6 Years

When children start school and their social world becomes increasingly rich, this provides further opportunities and challenges to developing self- and interpersonal understanding in the context of making new friends and finding their place in the social structure of the school. This also leads to better understanding of more complex social rules and dealing with issues of acceptance, inclusion, and exclusion.

With regard to their sense of self, the development of their autobiographical memory and its increasing sophistication around age 5 years also contributes to children's evolving capacity to describe themselves in terms of their own experiences and to begin to be able to give concrete examples (Music, 2011). By representing memories about the self and others more coherently and richly, children develop a sense of continuity, which in turn facilitates the development and integration of identity. At this age, children frequently describe themselves in terms of their abilities and tend to use comparisons with others (Harter, 2012; Nelson, 2003), but they might frequently find it difficult to distinguish between the superpowers that they wish to have and may have in fantasy and play (e.g., having magic rays that can freeze or shrink an enemy) and their real self, who, in fact, doesn't have these powers (Harter, 2012).

Age 6 to 7 Years

Six-year-olds have usually established the capacity to know what they and others will feel in different situations because the capacity for explicit mentalizing becomes established during the school years, building on the emotional understanding developed during the preschool period. However, during the early school years, children still need help from adults to explain and help them understand the reactions of others (e.g., when school friends react in ways that they don't understand and cause them distress due to exclusion, criticism, or being tricked). At the same time, they begin to develop the capacity to understand and make reference to emotions that require self-evaluation, such as pride, guilt, and shame (Thompson & Lagatutta, 2006). These also imply a certain awareness of social norms and expectations (Thompson, Meyer, & McGinley, 2006). They start to know that feelings can be disguised not to hurt the feelings of others, as when someone is disappointed with a gift (Weimer, Sallquist, & Bolnick, 2012).

At this age, children may begin to be able to use simple self-descriptions that capture something about their qualities, such as "I am kind and like to help," and they begin to be able to describe something about the quality of their close relationships.

Age 7 to 12 Years

At these ages, most children have developed sufficient cognitive sophistication to be able to think of themselves and others more in terms of individual personal qualities and mental states (Ensink, Target, Oandasan, & Duval, 2015), although for children at the lower end of this age group, this is generally simple, and they may struggle to find examples without some scaffolding.

As children progress through elementary school, mentalization rapidly becomes more sophisticated, enabling children to begin to see their own qualities in terms of what they are like as people and their personalities, and also to think about their attachment figures and describe their relationships in ways that capture the unique qualities that characterize these relationships (see Table 1.2). By this time, most normally developing children should have a well-established capacity to say what they feel and express complex and mixed emotions, as well as ambivalent feelings (Southam-Gerow & Kendall, 2002). They will have a well-developed understanding of a repertoire of more complicated interpersonal reactions built around previous experiences and explanations so that they only require help to understand interactions or situations that fall outside of this range.

From the age of 8 years, children become increasingly able to describe themselves in terms of personal characteristics such as *popular*, *helpful*, and *caring*, and they are able to capture something about themselves that remains stable across different contexts. Self-descriptions become more coherent, and autobiographical memories are more integrated with the particular experiences of the child. They begin to consider both positive and negative attributes of the self and to differentiate between the actual self and the self they wish to be (Harter, 2012), However, their growing self-awareness and capacity for self-evaluation also makes them more vulnerable and can have an impact on their self-esteem, and they may need help to integrate these observations in a way that can help them appreciate their strengths while acknowledging their weakness. At the same time, the capacity to see their own personalities and those of others helps them to increasingly make sense of interpersonal relations and understand the reactions of others who have personalities that are different from their own.

Finally, early adolescence is also an important period in the consolidation of identity and an awareness that one may have different selves expressed in different contexts (e.g., the self with one's parents differs from the self with friends). However, this change often comes without a child being able to recognize how these different aspects of the self are linked and what are the common unifying characteristics underlying them (Harter, 2012). For example, while a young adolescent may be quite outspoken and confident when with her parents, she may be shy and anxious when socializing with peers. However, she may not yet be able to clearly account for these differences and how this is linked to her sense of self. Later she may be able to do this, for example, saying, "I enjoy being around people, but I am not as extroverted as my friends and can get a little anxious when around a lot of people I don't know. I feel most at ease and confident when I am with people I know, like my family and close friends. Then I can actually be quite loud and funny at times."

CONCLUSION

In this chapter, we have introduced the notion of mentalizing and other key concepts, presented a theoretical model of the development of mentalizing in the contexts of reflective parenting, and described empirical evidence in support of this model. We have also illustrated what we mean by "good mentalizing" in the context of normal development. In the last part of this chapter, we have set out what we would expect mentalizing to look like in the course of normal development, from birth to age 12, and have specified the key developmental achievements in this regard as mentalizing unfolds. We hope that this developmental story will provide a helpful context for the clinical model that is described later in this book.

2

WHEN THE CAPACITY FOR MENTALIZING IS UNDERDEVELOPED OR BREAKS DOWN

In the previous chapter, we described how the capacity to mentalize develops throughout childhood and the role that mentalizing plays in the development of affect regulation, sense of self, and in supporting interpersonal relationships. We also explored the importance of reflective parenting in supporting children's development and looked at the ways in which infants, in the context of secure attachment relationships, can be helped to establish a curiosity about minds, which lays the foundation for epistemic trust and the capacity for social learning.

In this chapter, we turn to the ways in which mentalizing can go awry and the consequences this may have for children's development. We begin by stating clearly, however, that we do not believe all childhood emotional and behavioral problems are caused by mentalizing difficulties. Modern developmental psychopathology research shows that various interacting factors contribute to risk and resilience processes so that different roads lead to similar

http://dx.doi.org/10.1037/0000028-003
Mentalization-Based Treatment for Children: A Time-Limited Approach, by N. Midgley, K. Ensink, K. Lindqvist, N. Malberg, and N. Muller

psychological symptoms (Cicchetti & Rogosch, 1996; Schaffer, 2006). From this perspective, we see mentalizing as one of a number of important risk factors that need to be considered. However, we do believe that it is an important one to focus on not only because difficulties with mentalizing can be seen in a range of childhood disorders but also (and more important) because we believe that a focus on promoting mentalizing in therapy—both for parents and for children—may have significant clinical value. Whatever challenges and difficulties contribute to psychopathology, mentalizing, we argue, may be central in the process of potentially overcoming such difficulties, or at least living with them more adaptively.

A clear model is thus needed of how underdeveloped mentalizing, as well as mentalizing breakdowns and failures, may be implicated in a variety of psychological disorders. For this reason, we focus specifically on difficulties, deficits, and distortions in mentalizing as they relate to self and affect regulation—in relation to both children and their parents. In this chapter, we briefly outline our developmental model of breakdowns and failures in mentalizing before presenting in more detail how this is connected with the kind of difficulties that often bring children to the attention of psychological services.

A FRAMEWORK FOR THINKING ABOUT MENTALIZING DIFFICULTIES

First of all, we want to be clear that difficulties or breakdowns in mentalizing are perfectly normal and occur all the time, so there is nothing inherently pathological when we speak about problems with mentalizing. It is an inevitable part of human interactions that we misread people's intentions or make attributions that later turn out to be wrong. Research has suggested that from the age of 3 months onward, infants look for a "high but imperfect" level of contingent response from their caregiver and that it is not necessarily helpful for parents to be too perfect in their capacity to read their child's mind (Gergely & Watson, 1999). Fonagy (2015) quoted the work of Tronick (2007) approvingly when he noted that "miscommunication and 'messiness' lie at the heart of the development of the self and self-regulation. Miscommunication creates negative affect, but, when interactive errors are repaired, the negative is replaced by positive affect in both infant and mother" (p. 361). It is no accident that "understanding mis-understanding" is one of the most important definitions of mentalizing because misreading the intention of others, then recognizing this and repairing it, is a crucial element of all lasting relationships.

Furthermore, our capacity for mentalizing is a fragile one, liable to break down at least temporarily, especially when we are under stress or in a state of emotional arousal. We would probably all recognize some of the ways in which our capacity to reflect on the mental states of self and other become far more limited when we are highly stressed; this is both normal and expected. Nevertheless, in a certain respect, difficulties and breakdowns in mentalizing can create problems for both parents and children. Sometimes we may simply be faced with challenges we haven't encountered before, such as a sudden loss or a difficult situation with peers. In such situations, ordinary or even good mentalizing that has been developed to deal with everyday situations may not be enough. An analogy here could be that of a pilot who knows how to fly a small plane but will be at risk when flying in a storm without specific knowledge about the storm winds raging in a specific area and without particular skills in being able to fly based on the radar only.

In general terms, mentalizing difficulties can be considered from two broad perspectives. On the one hand, we can think of problems arising from an *underdeveloped mentalizing capacity*. Many children (and some adults) may have limited capacity to know what they are feeling and then use this understanding to guide self and affect regulation. For example, they may show little capacity to think about themselves and relationships in mental state terms or may describe themselves and others only in physical and behavioral terms. In such cases, there may be a therapeutic benefit in helping to build or better establish a capacity for mentalizing, or, in some cases, to focus on supporting the "building blocks" of mentalizing and self- and affect regulation, including a capacity for attention control (Fonagy, Gergely, Jurist, & Target, 2002; Fonagy & Target, 2006).

There are times, however, when difficulties may be more clearly associated with a *breakdown of mentalizing*, either temporary and context specific or more chronic (see Table 2.1). Often this may take the form of a switch away from more controlled, explicit mentalizing, usually in the context of heightened emotional states of stress or arousal. From an evolutionary perspective, this switching makes good sense because explicit mentalizing relies on slower neural processes and a capacity for effortful control. A switch to more automatic forms of mentalizing is quicker but less accurate and may take the form of what Bateman and Fonagy (2009) have referred to as prementalistic or nonmentalizing modes of experiencing the self and others. These are described in more detail later in the chapter.

WHEN PARENTS STRUGGLE TO MENTALIZE

However good our capacity to mentalize may be under normal circumstances, there is no doubt that family life and being a parent place huge strains on our capacity to mentalize. Fonagy and Allison (2012) wrote that

TABLE 2.1
Underdeveloped Mentalizing Versus Specific Mentalizing
Difficulties and Breakdowns

Underdeveloped	Breakdowns and difficulties
These children have ongoing deficits in mentalizing.	Emotional or behavioral difficulties occur for these children in the context of an established basic capacity for mentalizing.
These children may be unaware of how they are reacting or have limited capacity to identify feelings and express them verbally. They struggle to consider the feelings and intentions of others, to understand their behavior, and to predict their reactions.	These children have age-appropriate abilities to think about their reactions and those of others in terms of underlying feelings and motivations.
These children may have difficulty with self-regulation and find it difficult to be aware of their reactions and those of others.	These children are able to self-regulate at a level expected for their age, express feelings and thoughts about themselves and others, and can use this knowledge to understand interpersonal reactions. This ability may be lost when distressed or angry or when overwhelmed by difficult experiences or situations.
Affects may be acted out physically or behaviorally, and these children have little ability to reflect about this or put the experience into words. Not knowing what they feel, or being unaware of the impact of their actions on others, leaves them unable to use explicit mentalizing to modulate their reactions and contain affects.	These children may be unable to express and think about certain feelings, or struggle with contradictory or "unacceptable" feelings. They may lose their capacity to mentalize when overwhelmed, afraid, or angry, or they may need help to elaborate their reactions in the context of a safe relationship.
These children may have no clear sense of self and their attributes, abilities, and weaknesses. Others are often seen only in terms of current behavior and utility and whether they are a source of frustration or gratification.	These children have a sense of self, their personalities, and who they are and can see others in terms of both their good and bad qualities. They are able to relate to others appropriately, although there may be difficulties in some specific contexts or with specific people.

there is no context more likely to induce a loss of mentalizing than family interactions. It is within the family that relationships tend to be at their most fraught, their most loving and their most intense emotionally; in other words, the family is an environment with the potential to stimulate a loss of mentalizing in one or more members of the family, on a daily basis. (p. 24)

Even parents who are generally sensitive may not be able to know how to guide their children when they are faced with really difficult situations. Mentalization may break down when parents are overwhelmed with financial or other difficulties or are faced with challenges such as immigration or divorce; in such stressful and overwhelming contexts, they may not be able to keep their children in mind or be emotionally available for them or may struggle much more to do so. Parents who have more chronic difficulties with mentalizing may well have had parents who in turn were not reflective in their style of parenting, even if their childhood was not overtly abusive or traumatic. For example, their own parents might have given them the message that "crying is for babies" and that sad or vulnerable feelings should be either ignored or mastered. On becoming parents themselves, it may in turn be difficult for these parents to tolerate or actively mirror their own infant's more vulnerable feelings.

In *Anna Karenina*, Tolstoy wrote, "All happy families are alike; each unhappy family is unhappy in its own way." Likewise, Bateman and Fonagy (2016) noted that although "good mentalizing takes just one form, non-mentalizing may be indicated by a wide range of possible manifestations" (p. 66). When parents are struggling to mentalize, it may appear in a number of ways, such as the following:

- a focus on their child's behavior, without attention to their mental states or internal experience;
- excessive blaming or fault-finding;
- trying to control their child's behavior, through authoritarian styles of parenting (Baumrind, 1966);
- exhibiting unmodulated mental states themselves, without awareness of the impact these may have on their child; and/or
- demonstrating negative distortions and attributions to their child (e.g., asserting that their child is crying "because she wants to punish me").

At times parents struggle to see beyond children's behaviors and consider the feelings underlying them. In those circumstances, they may not be able to see the child's distress and may react to the child's behavior in ways that are likely to escalate them rather than help the child feel understood. At times like this, parents and their children may get into *nonmentalizing vicious cycles* in which a powerful emotion in one family member may reduce their capacity to mentalize, which in turn makes it harder for them to understand the other's behavior or intentions. Figure 2.1 illustrates such a vicious cycle, in which Person 1's powerful emotions lead him to temporarily lose his capacity for mentalizing, so that he struggles to understand the intentions or feelings of the other person. This can then make the other person's behavior seem incomprehensible, which can in turn trigger an attempt to try and control the other person. Such controlling behavior can be frightening or distressing for the other person, which therefore creates powerful emotions in Person 2. The same cycle of responses is then triggered in her, leading to a vicious cycle of nonmentalizing interactions. For example, when a child is upset, she may think that her father's attempt to calm her down is "just trying to make me be quiet" (misreading of her father's intention). This in turn can lead the child to become more controlling in her behavior, for example, by kicking or pushing her dad away. This may create distress and heightened emotional arousal in the girl's father because people do not like feeling misunderstood, and when this happens, it can create powerful feelings of hostility and rejection. The girl's father may thus become less mentalizing and less well-equipped to reflect on his daughter's behavior. For example, the father, in his frustration, may think "she's just doing this to be difficult because she knows I need to cook supper," and this misattribution will in turn make him behave in a more controlling way, shouting at his daughter or telling her, "That's it then, no television today!" This controlling behavior is likely to make his daughter

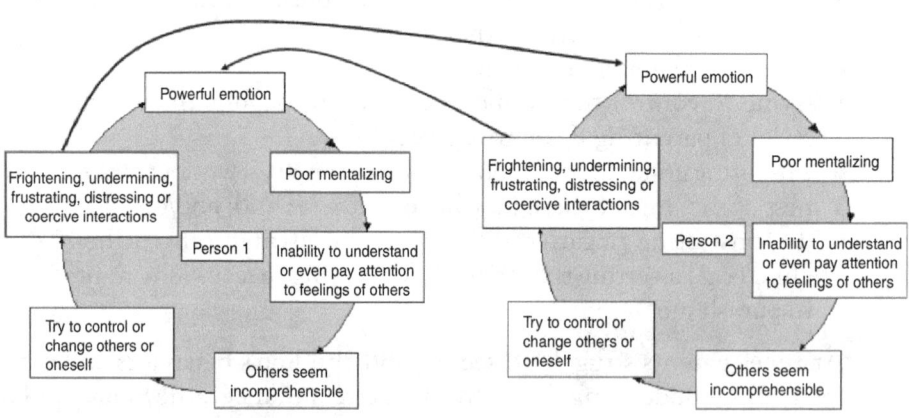

Figure 2.1. The vicious cycles of mentalizing problems in families. From *Handbook of Mentalization-Based Treatment* (p. 208), by J. G. Allen and P. Fonagy (Eds.), 2006, Chichester, England: John Wiley & Sons. Copyright 2008 by John Wiley & Sons. Adapted with permission.

more angry and upset, thereby increasing her emotional arousal and reducing her capacity to mentalize. And so the vicious cycle continues.

In other circumstances, there may be various reasons why a parent may struggle to maintain a reflective capacity in relation to his or her child. When parents are immature, substance abusing, or prone to dissociation, they may psychologically withdraw from their children and not engage in the interactions and communication essential to help them develop their own mentalizing capacities. Some parents with difficult temperaments may be good at mentalizing when not emotionally activated but may be unable to step back and see themselves from the outside when they lose control, and so they fail to see the impact of their own behavior. The bottom line is that parents with difficult temperaments need to be particularly adept at mentalizing about themselves to help them to gain perspective and develop strategies to protect their children and modulate their own aggression.

Serious failures in parental mentalizing are sometimes associated with parental mental illness, personality disorder, or unresolved trauma in the parent's own history. Mentalization regarding trauma is particularly challenging, and failures in mentalizing about trauma and its impact on one's development, personality, and parenting leave people particularly vulnerable to failures in monitoring and modulating inappropriate trauma-related affects in relationships with partners and children (Berthelot, Ensink, et al., 2015; Ensink, Berthelot, Bernazzani, Normandin, & Fonagy, 2014). For these parents, mentalization may be so distorted that they are constantly in a state in which they are sure that what is in their own mind is what the child is really feeling or thinking. Some parents may not be particularly reflective about themselves and may not be aware when they are aggressive, especially when it is a reaction to anxiety or fear or when it is linked to personality or trauma.

As the literature on mentalization has expanded, a broad range of nonmentalizing styles have been identified. For example, some parents talk about the problems of their child by only focusing on behavior and describing what is physically observable. This has been described as *concrete mentalizing* and reflects a general failure to appreciate that internal states can provide a way to understand behavior. Parents functioning in this way may display no curiosity as to what the behavior of their child could say about their feelings, wishes, or needs. Often emphasis is placed on external social factors such as school or the neighborhood. The behavior of the child may be explained in terms of "he was born this way" or "this is just the way he is," and labels such as "he is an ADHD child" might be used as explanation. Phrases such as "he always . . ." or "she never . . ." are cues that a parent may be short-circuiting the process of trying to understand his or her child's behavior and instead relying on fixed explanations. This often has a blaming quality rather than exhibiting true acceptance of the child's individual qualities or a potentially important understanding of something central about the child's nature.

In other situations, parents who at times can be thoughtful and reflective about their child's experience may suddenly shift when faced with certain situations. Such *context-specific loss of mentalizing* may be because their child's behavior has been a trigger that inhibits their own capacity for mentalization. For instance, consider a mother who has a history of sexual abuse and does not want her daughter to stay overnight at her friend's house because she fears her daughter might be sexually assaulted. In this situation, depending on the age of the child and who intervenes, it is not surprising that this mother might find it difficult to differentiate her need to protect out of fear and her child's need for peer interaction. To her daughter, who may not be able to understand the intention behind her mother's behavior, she may come across as insensitive and rigid.

UNDERDEVELOPED MENTALIZING IN CHILDREN

Some of the children who are referred to child mental health services may have a limited capacity to mentalize about themselves or others, evidenced by their being unable to know what they feel and unable to use reflections on feeling states to facilitate self- and affect regulation. Indications that such children are likely to have an underdeveloped capacity to mentalize may be when they

- do not know and cannot identify what they are feeling;
- cannot use knowledge of affects to self-regulate;
- cannot see themselves from outside (e.g., how angry they are);
- cannot identify their reactions to hurt, sadness, fear, and anger;
- cannot describe what they are like as people (i.e., their personality);
- cannot tell a story of their lives (i.e., their autobiography);
- demonstrate difficulties related to extreme temperament; and/or
- ruminate (i.e., have difficulties with thinking too much).

In some cases, this underdeveloped capacity for mentalizing may be primarily attributable to genetics. For example, children with autistic spectrum disorder (ASD) may have limitations in basic mentalizing abilities that others take for granted, such as the ability to read the minds of others by analyzing their facial expressions. In most cases, individuals with ASD may not be able to develop automatic empathy, intuitively consider the needs of others, or be able to see themselves from the outside and consider the impact of their own behavior on others (Frith, 2004). To compensate for these deficits in implicit mentalizing, they often develop explicit mentalizing strategies over time, but painfully and sometimes with little help from others.

Other children who are brought for psychological help may not have had sufficient help and opportunity to develop representations of themselves in terms of personal characteristics and personality. This can contribute to difficulties in the capacity to see themselves through others' eyes and think about the impact their behavior has on others. Not having a basic sense of themselves, in terms of what they and their personalities are like, also makes it difficult for these children to make choices that are well-matched to their personal qualities and abilities, which will help them build on their strengths and develop them further.

Many children who are referred for help have few opportunities to learn to identify what they are feeling and to express this when they are in pain, afraid, or want something. Children growing up with parents who struggle to take a reflective stance, are behaviorally focused, and punish behaviors they consider problematic, have few opportunities to learn to think about themselves and their behaviors as being motivated by underlying mental states. Without a parent with whom the child can reflect on experiences (e.g., rejection or teasing by a group at school), few children are able to develop a more nuanced mental-state understanding on their own. These children may not have had the opportunities to learn and develop basic capacities to identify their own feelings and be aware of their own reactions and their impact on others, or to understand the feelings and motivations that may underlie the reactions of others. They may have difficulty noticing the intentions of others and have insufficiently elaborated or unbalanced mental representations of self and others. For example, when a teacher reacts with anger when provoked, children with underdeveloped mentalizing may only be able to see the reaction of the teacher and may react as if the teacher is nasty and they are being unfairly victimized, without considering how they have provoked the teacher who is normally patient and tolerant. These children also frequently have difficulties with affect regulation, poor social capacities, and weak attention regulation. They are likely to have an insecure or disorganized attachment style (Fonagy, Gergely, Jurist, & Target, 2002), and there is sometimes a history of neglect or trauma.

Children who grow up with parents with psychiatric disorders or substance abuse that have affected their capacities to parent, or children who are traumatized, adopted, or in foster care, frequently have underdeveloped mentalizing capacities. This is because the multiple processes through which children develop these abilities have been negatively influenced by the ongoing experiences of neglect, disruption, and maltreatment (Ostler, Bahar, & Jessee, 2010).

For children with particularly sensitive, fearful, or difficult temperaments or personalities, it may be especially important to develop the capacity to see themselves from the outside with a benign and playful regard that will help them understand their strengths, but also their challenges. Ordinary mentalizing may not be enough, and ideally the parents of these children need to be more reflective than other parents to help their child understand why others might react to them in certain ways. Children with temperamentally based extreme fearfulness (Kochanska, Aksan, & Joy, 2007), anxiousness (Lengua, 2008), or sensory processing sensitivity (Aron, Aron, & Davies, 2005) may need additional help from reflective parents (or therapists) and may be vulnerable when parents are unable to adjust their parenting based on an empathic understanding of the child's psychological experience. A reflective stance may be particularly important for parents to understand and respond in ways that are sensitive to the specific challenges these children face.

Some children, with or without histories of abuse, have extreme difficulties with affect regulation because of their temperamental sensitivity. For example, a child in a special school might regularly be sent to a "quiet room" (isolation) when he becomes dysregulated because this is the only way the school can think of to try to help him regain regulation. However, these sanctions probably contribute to him becoming even more disorganized. Children with temperaments like this, where they have more negative affectivity, impulsivity, or aggression, need to be better than other children at mentalizing about themselves and the impact of their behavior on others if they are to modulate their negative behavior and limit damage to interpersonal relationships. There is evidence suggesting that in low-risk contexts, preschoolers with more impulsive aggression learn to know more about aggression and its impact on others than children with easy temperaments and that this knowledge is related to whether they are liked or rejected despite their aggression (Laurent & Ensink, 2016).

DIFFERENT MODES OF NONMENTALIZING IN CHILDREN

Having described various ways in which children may have an underdeveloped capacity to mentalize, we now turn to the various modes of nonmentalizing that clinicians and researchers working in this field have identified. In their work on understanding and treating adults with borderline personality disorder (BPD), Bateman and Fonagy (2004) began by noticing a set of key deficits that were characteristic of this particular disorder: impulsiveness, difficulties with emotional regulation, relationship problems, and problems of identity formation. In their seminal work on BPD, they argued that all of these difficulties could be understood as a result of difficulties with mentalizing, in particular, in perceiving the mental states of self and others with sufficient accuracy. On the basis of their clinical experience with such patients, they identified certain patterns of pre- or nonmentalizing thinking, which seemed to be activated in their patients when in a state of stress or tension or when the attachment system was highly aroused, as was often the case when forming a therapeutic relationship.

Bateman and Fonagy (2004) went on to describe three typical patterns or modes of nonmentalizing, which they hypothesized may be part of normal development but for most people are rapidly replaced by a more mature capacity for slow and reflective mentalizing. They named these modes the teleological, psychic equivalence, and pretend modes. Although these modes were identified in the context of work with adults with BPD, we believe that they can be of help when working with mentalizing difficulties in children and parents, so we introduce each of them briefly here.

In the *teleological mode* (which, because the word is rather technical, we sometimes simply refer to as "quick-fix thinking"), "changes in mental states are assumed to be real only when confirmed by physically observable action contingent upon the patient's wish, belief, feeling or desire" (Bateman & Fonagy, 2016, p. 23). In other words, when operating in a teleological mode, only an immediate action seems like a possible solution and is thus aggressively or anxiously demanded, much like when a baby cries action may be called for and only immediate feeding or a diaper change will suffice. Although this immediate response and action may be appropriate in the contexts of taking care of babies, later in development the assumption that action is needed, or interpersonal difficulties or distress can only be solved through action, can be problematic. Rather than having a notion of feelings in the self that can be thought about, understood, and resolved, there is a conviction that mental states can only be "solved" by means of physical action. When someone is operating in a teleological mode, a quick solution or specific actions are demanded, and there is a refusal to consider mental states underlying behaviors. So when a child says, "When my mom gives me money, that's how I know she loves me" or a parent says, "The only solution is for my son to be on Ritalin," then they may be operating in a nonmentalizing, teleological way.

In the *psychic equivalent mode* (which can more simply be described as "inside-out thinking"), the perception of external reality is distorted by internal states; there is no interest in internal states in the self or in others, and any attempt to draw attention to them may be angrily rejected. The child may be convinced that others always get preferential treatment, and he is unfairly treated; and because that is what he thinks, he sees it as a fact. In younger children, this may be developmentally appropriate (e.g., if a young child imagines that there may be a monster under the bed, she may believe there really is a monster there), in older children (or adults), this kind of "mind–world isomorphism" makes it difficult for the person to take another perspective or to see his or her thoughts as something that can be explored and thought about or treated with curiosity. In extreme cases (as in BPD), this may take the form of "rigid inflexible thought processes, inappropriate conviction of being right, extravagant claims of knowing what is on someone else's mind or why certain actions were performed" (Bateman & Fonagy, 2016, p. 21). As most parents will recognize, however, this description is fairly recognizable from arguments with a typical teenager, which only confirms that all of us are likely to fall into nonmentalizing ways of thinking under stressful circumstances.

The third form of prementalistic thinking that Bateman and Fonagy (2016) described is the *pretend mode* (or what we might call "elephant-in-the-room thinking"). When operating in this mode, there is "a separation between psychic and physical activity to a point where the connection between the two can no longer be achieved" (pp. 21–22). When the mental world is decoupled from reality and becomes more real than reality, this interferes with and undermines normal development. Children operating in pretend mode may even use a lot of mental-state language but without this being meaningfully linked to their reality (e.g., having grandiose and self-serving descriptions of their abilities and plans and how much others admire them, but not engaging with the real issues of their failing grades or risking expulsion from school for bullying). With parents, the pretend mode can sometimes leave the listener with a sense that there has been endless inconsequential talk about thoughts and feelings but without any genuine quality. Often it is an indication that something else may be going on, which is not being sufficiently attended to (hence, the elephant in the room).

Pretend mode is also the favored mode of nonmentalizing for some therapists and can usually be spotted when we find ourselves using clever and internally coherent words that have no connection to the actual feeling states of the people in the room. As with most nonmentalizing modes, we are most likely to fall into this when we are anxious or stressed (e.g., when feeling that we need to come up with a clever response when faced with an angry parent demanding that we make the situation better), and as with all nonmentalizing modes, the first step in addressing it in others or in ourselves is to notice it.

ATTACHMENT AND BREAKS IN MENTALIZING

As we have tried to emphasize throughout this chapter, not all childhood psychopathology, and not all difficulties with mentalizing, can be traced back to the early parent–child relationship. Severe autism is a case in point: Even the most loving parenting cannot resolve the many severe difficulties these children present with, and parents need all the help and support they can get to continue dealing with the challenges of providing loving care in difficult circumstances. In addition, we know little about children at the far end of the spectrum of temperament, who display extreme reactivity, impulsivity, or hypersensitivity, and to what extent parental care can be effective in modulating these vulnerability factors over time.

Nevertheless, in many cases, early childhood experiences are important, and an attachment perspective can provide us with a clinical tool that is useful for understanding certain kinds of mentalizing breakdowns. It also helps to understand how strong feelings or stress in parents and children can trigger dramatic breakdowns in mentalizing, even in individuals who can be reflective at other times.

As we set out in the previous chapter, when children are *securely attached*, they are more likely to see their caregivers as reliable sources of knowledge and to show curiosity about mental states in themselves and others. These children are more likely to accurately read the intentions of others and to show empathy and emotional attunement. In their relationships with others, they are often better at resolving conflict situations because they are able to make use of their perspective-taking skills to see the views of others and to regulate their own affects by using explicit, controlled mentalizing. Secure attachment facilitates mentalizing and can be seen as organizing the brain in a way that promotes social cooperation and strong relationships (Fonagy, 2015). This is not to say that children (or adults) with a secure attachment are not vulnerable to mentalizing breakdowns; rather, in most cases, these children will be able to recover their capacity to mentalize relatively quickly and use it to effectively down-regulate their stress levels. As Luyten and Fonagy (2015) put it, individuals who predominantly use secure attachment strategies when faced with adversity "have the ability to turn to (internalized) secure attachment figures in times of need, they find interpersonal contacts rewarding, and they have the capacity to keep controlled mentalizing 'online' even when faced with considerable stress" (p. 373).

For children with more insecure attachment patterns, the picture is different (Taylor, 2012). Children with *insecure avoidant* (or *dismissive*) *attachment* styles have learned to use deactivating strategies in which they minimize and deny attachment needs and dependency, as well as their feelings. They generally show avoidance of mentalizing about relationships and low mentalization regarding others, taking a cognitive route to thinking about relationships that may be disconnected from affect. This can often present as undermentalizing—that is, children give a reduced mental-state account of events, and the emotional impact of interpersonal behaviors is not considered. In such cases, children may simply seem not to pay attention to what others think or show a lack of interest in what others feel about them. They may emphasize their own independence, working on the belief that others cannot provide support or comfort to them.

In some respects, children with avoidant attachment states of mind may look like those with more secure forms of attachment with regard to mentalizing. They may be able to think about others' mental states and also, to some extent, their own because attachment deactivation strategies allow controlled mentalizing to stay "online" (Vrticka, Andersson, Grandjean, Sander, & Vuilleumier, 2008). However, this mentalizing will often be overly cognitive and can sometimes have the quality of pretend-mode thinking, with their words lacking emotional resonance. Furthermore, in situations of high stress, these children may not be able to recover their mentalizing capacity in the way that more securely children can usually do, leaving them overwhelmed by affect (Mikulincer & Shaver, 2007).

Children with *insecure preoccupied* (or *ambivalent*) *attachment styles* are also at a particularly elevated risk for psychological difficulties, so it is clinically useful to be aware how this tends to present. Whereas children with an insecure-avoidant attachment style have learned to use *deactivating* strategies to minimize and deny attachment needs and dependency, these children are more likely to use attachment *hyperactivating* strategies. This means that they have a fairly low threshold, when faced with stressful situations, for switching from more controlled, reflective mentalizing into nonmentalizing modes and become dependent on others to regulate them (Fonagy, Luyten, Allison, & Campbell, 2016).

When asked to think about attachment relationships, as in the Child Attachment Interview (Target, Fonagy, & Shmueli-Goetz, 2003), these children often focus on the failings of others but are unable to "finish the story," as if mentalizing cannot contain the emotion. Instead, preoccupied anger drives an endless unsuccessful search for alternative mental solutions. In structured attachment interviews, this is evident in long, rambling narratives that are difficult to follow and where there may be a great deal of pseudo-mentalizing, but the listener ends up feeling confused. These children usually understand that there are feelings and thoughts behind people's actions, but they are likely to misunderstand both, leading to inaccurate assumptions about other people and their intentions (Taylor, 2012). When asked to describe situations with a parent, such children often seem unwilling to think of why the parent may have behaved in a certain way, even when it is evident to the listener, or, alternatively, they may be unable to wrap things up mentally by saying, for example, "I don't know why my mom behaved that way," rather than trying to reflect or becoming curious.

Preoccupied attachment styles are relatively rare in low-risk populations but more common in children with histories of abuse and neglect, and also in youth with emerging personality disorder (Rosenstein & Horowitz, 1996). In the context of abuse and neglect, preoccupied styles (compared with avoidant styles) are costly in terms of functioning because these children remain emotionally entangled and focused on a parent whose behavior they are unlikely to change or understand, and this interferes with self- and affect-regulation. These children can sometimes come across as controlling or manipulative, which in turn reduces the likelihood that the adults around them will respond in a reflective way.

In children who have *disorganized attachment styles*, we often observe a complete breakdown of mentalization under stress, just at the moments when they are most in need of their mentalizing capacities. These children often show features of both hypermentalizing and catastrophic breakdowns in mentalizing, which are also seen in young people with emerging personality disorder (Fonagy, Luyten, Allison, & Campbell, 2016). Drawing on his extensive clinical experience with children in foster care, Taylor (2012) carefully described how children with disorganized attachment styles, as they reach school age, may make superficial judgments about other people based on how they appear and have little capacity for perspective-taking. For these children, interpersonal stress, such as conflict, rejection, or criticism, can easily activate disorganized states—especially in attachment relationships, but also when facing apparently simple challenges that may be experienced as overwhelming. So when asked if he will help set the table, a child with a disorganized attachment may react with fury because he misread this request as a criticism that he does not help enough around the house. Such violent reactions can in turn challenge the caregiver's capacity to remain reflective, leading to the kind of nonmentalizing vicious cycles described earlier in the chapter.

Whereas children with secure attachment styles are able to maintain mentalizing or rapidly regain their ability to regulate, children with disorganized attachment lack strategies for regaining regulation when they become distressed. This may be linked to earlier experiences in which, when distressed as an infant, the parents failed to respond or responded in ways that increased, rather than decreased, the infant's distress, thus undermining the development of organized strategies for regaining and achieving self- and affect regulation. Failures to respond to infant distress are most apparent in contexts of abuse and neglect, where parents manifest extreme withdrawal so that the infant may be left for long periods in states of distress or where parents react in ways that induce fear (e.g., by becoming angry and aggressive). However, attachment disorganization is also observed in low-risk mother–infant dyads where it has been linked to a history of unresolved loss and trauma in the parent and where the infant's distress triggers trauma-related affects so that the mother reacts with fear or shows fear-inducing behaviors.

Berthelot, Ensink, Bernazzani, Normandin, Luyten, and Fonagy (2015) have proposed that risks associated with disorganized attachment can be understood in terms of a failure in parental mentalizing and marked affect mirroring. In early infancy, caregivers may have responded with their own trauma-related affects completely disconnected to the infant, rather than responding sensitively to the infant's distress. This is thought to leave the infant with a sense of being trapped with distress that cannot be related to and thus with a desperate sense of being "bad" and totally alone or abandoned when they are at their most distressed and most in need of help. These experiences of unmetabolized distress can lead to experiences of incoherence of the self that are so painful, they trigger dissociation or acting out.

It is argued that the kind of attachment strategies children use may have implications for their capacity for epistemic trust. Children who are securely attached are more likely to have confidence in their own experience, so that they are both able to learn from trusted adults and to know when to trust their own judgment. An anxious attachment is more likely to create a sense of epistemic uncertainty ("Is it safe to learn from this person and have confidence in what she says?"), whereas an avoidant attachment may be more associated with epistemic mistrust ("I don't think it is safe to believe what the other person is teaching me."). For disorganized attachment, there is an even greater extreme, epistemic *hypervigilance*, which is based on the unresolvable question "Who can I trust?" (Fonagy & Allison, 2014, p. 374). These children may even mistrust their own experience. This can lay the groundwork for a potentially interminable epistemic search in which such children seek others to confirm or deny their own understanding and feeling, yet find it impossible to trust the information once it has been received. The implications of this for assessment and therapy are explored in later chapters of this book.

FAILURES IN MENTALIZING RELATED TO ABUSE AND NEGLECT

Trauma, especially relational trauma in the context of early abuse and neglect, is recognized as a key factor increasing the risk for all types of psychiatric disorders (Cicchetti & Banny, 2014; Dorahy, Middleton, Seager, Williams, & Chambers, 2016; Dvir, Ford, Hill, & Frazier, 2014). This appears to be the case for depressive and anxiety disorders, as well as personality disorders such as BPD, but also for psychotic disorders such as schizophrenia, which until recently was considered primarily genetically determined (Berthelot, Paccalet, et al., 2015). Early trauma, such as child abuse and neglect, as well as harsh or affectionless parenting, is considered an important stress factor that undermines and disrupts normal development of self- and affect regulation and act as a general diathesis that can activate underlying genetic risks for psychopathology.

In addition, specific types of abuse, such as attachment or betrayal trauma (Allen, 2008; Freyd & Birrell, 2013), in which a child has been abused by an attachment figure that should have been a source of protection and security, are known to have especially negative consequences in terms of undermining trust. Such experiences profoundly disrupt development because they leave children with the sense that others cannot be trusted, learned from, or confided in when in trouble or in distress. At the same time, their attachment systems may be permanently activated by a sense of fear and distress, leaving these children with few self-regulation strategies.

Children who have experienced attachment trauma and grow up in contexts of abuse and neglect frequently present with underdeveloped capacities to think about themselves and others. They also tend to focus mainly on behavior and use automatic modes of mentalizing adapted to detect threat and need help developing slower, more reflective mentalizing. They frequently have an underdeveloped capacity to know what they feel and how to use this knowledge to facilitate self-regulation (Ostler et al., 2010).

We believe that mentalizing is especially vulnerable to *relational trauma*, that is, trauma or abuse that happens in the context of primary relationships (Allen, Lemma, & Fonagy, 2012). It is proposed that children growing up in a context in which caregivers cannot be trusted adapt by constantly being in a state of hypervigilance (Ensink, Berthelot, et al., 2014; Fonagy & Allison, 2014). As a result, they become closed to the minds of others, in contrast to the normal curiosity of children about the motivations and intentions of others. Furthermore, they habitually use automatic modes of mentalizing that are predominantly concerned with detection of threats to survival, so it becomes increasingly difficult to break this pattern and engage in more reflective, explicit mentalizing (Ensink, Bégin, Normandin, Godbout, & Fonagy, 2016). Children may actively avoid mentalization to protect an attachment relationship or because they fear to think about the (possibly malevolent) intentions of others.

Maltreated children manifest a range of sociocognitive and mentalizing deficits (Cicchetti, Rogosch, Maughan, Toth, & Bruce, 2003; Ensink, Normandin, et al., 2015; Pears & Fisher, 2005), including difficulties in thinking about themselves and attachment relationships in mental-state terms. This has been associated with depressive as well as externalizing symptoms (Ensink, Bégin, Normandin, & Fonagy, 2016). Young maltreated children elaborate and complete fewer play narratives than other children; interestingly, the capacity to elaborate play narratives predicts their later mentalization capacities and mediates the relationship between abuse and mentalization (Tessier, Normandin, Ensink, & Fonagy, 2016). Maltreated children also engage in less symbolic play and are less likely to initiate dyadic play (Valentino, Cicchetti, Toth, & Rogosch, 2011). They make fewer references to their internal mental states (Shipman & Zeman, 1999), struggle to understand emotions expressed in faces, and are less likely to express empathy when other children are in distress (Klimes-Dougan & Kistner, 1990).

Furthermore, in the context of abuse, low mentalization appears to further increase the risk of dissociation in children (Ensink, Bégin, Normandin, Godbout, & Fonagy, 2016). Maltreated children are particularly vulnerable to dissociation (Macfie, Cicchetti, & Toth, 2001) because processes that contribute to metacognitive integration and mental-state understanding, such as the capacity to suspend reality in the context of pretend play, may also contribute to dissociation (Putnam, 1997; Wieland & Silberg, 2013). Because dissociation undermines the development of strategies for tolerating and integrating affect and thinking about the consequences of actions (Fonagy, 2004), dissociation increases the risk of manifesting maladapted behaviors.

MENTALIZING DIFFICULTIES AND CHILDHOOD DISORDERS

Many researchers and clinicians have strong views on the value (or lack of value) of psychiatric diagnosis when trying to make sense of the mental health of children (e.g., Timimi, 2002). In the context of mentalization theory, Fonagy and Campbell (2015) noted the limited explanatory power of more descriptive, category-driven approaches to psychopathology. They pointed out that in a longitudinal study by Caspi et al. (2014) that examined the structure of psychopathology from adolescence through to adulthood, psychiatric disorders were best explained by one general psychopathology factor, which the authors called the *p factor*. Fonagy and Campbell suggested that this mysterious but determining p factor may turn out to be epistemic trust and speculated that "an individual with a high p factor score [which predicts greater lifetime risk of a range of psychopathologies] is one in a state of epistemic hypervigilance and epistemic mistrust" (p. 243). Although such lines of enquiry are intriguing, in this section, we take a more conservative position and describe what the empirical research suggests so far about the role of mentalizing difficulties in various psychiatric disorders in children. This knowledge is inevitably tentative but expanding rapidly.

As indicated earlier, difficulties with mentalizing may contribute to a wide range of childhood disorders, and strengthening mentalization can therefore have a positive effect for children presenting with diverse symptoms or behaviors. This is not to say, however, that all childhood mental health difficulties should be thought of as "mentalizing disorders" in the way that could be argued, for instance, in the case of BPD (Fonagy & Bateman, 2007). What is presented here is only a snapshot, but the literature has been reviewed in more detail elsewhere (e.g., Ensink, Bégin, Normandin, & Fonagy, 2016; Ensink & Mayes, 2010; Sharp, Fonagy, & Goodyer, 2008; Sharp & Venta, 2012).

Much of the original impetus for examining the role of mentalizing in childhood disorders came about as a result of the increasing interest in understanding ASD. Most of the empirical research in this area draws on a narrower, more cognitive idea of mentalizing—in particular, theory of mind (see Chapter 1, this volume). Baron-Cohen, Leslie, and Frith (1985) were the first to suggest that children with autism were less able to pass the false-belief task than age-matched children either with Down syndrome or who were normally developing. On this basis, Baron-Cohen et al. postulated that children with ASD suffer from "mind-blindness." Subsequent research has suggested that the picture is less black-and-white than was first suggested, and in his later work (e.g., Baron-Cohen, 2009), Baron-Cohen has suggested that all children are on an "empathizing continuum," and children with ASD are usually at the lower end of this spectrum. In reviewing a considerable body of empirical work in this area, Sharp and Venta (2012) concluded that "a solid body of literature suggests reduced mentalizing capacity in autistic children and adolescents across all developmental stages" (p. 38).

The picture is less clear-cut with the other common childhood disorders, including the internalizing disorders, such an anxiety and depression. There is evidence that lower understanding of emotions and strategies to hide and change emotions (Southam-Gerow & Kendall, 2002) are associated with an increased risk of anxiety disorders, although not all anxious children have mentalization difficulties. In reviewing research on anxiety disorders, Sharp and Venta (2012) quoted Banerjee (2008) in concluding that there is now a substantial amount of empirical evidence to support the view that anxious youth experience "difficulty with understanding and effectively managing social situations involving multiple mental states" (p. 253). These difficulties may be associated with both the social skills deficits and hypervigilance with regard to the minds of others that are features of anxiety. On the basis of clinical experience, and given the links between emotional dysregulation and mentalizing, it is easy to imagine that when children's baseline anxiety is high, it takes little additional arousal to push them over the edge into nonmentalizing (Haslam-Hopwood, Allen, Stein, & Bleiberg, 2006). Although breakdowns in mentalizing may not be the cause of anxiety, it is easy to imagine that helping children become better able to recognize their triggers for overarousal and anxiety states could be one benefit of a better capacity to mentalize for those suffering from anxiety.

Like many early-life stressors, trauma and intrapersonal conflicts may contribute to depression in childhood, and children's mentalizing about themselves and others appears to be an important potential resource in the context of depressive symptoms. There is evidence that by age 7 to 12, children's mentalizing about themselves and attachment figures is inversely associated with depressive symptoms (Ensink, Bégin, Normandin, & Fonagy, 2016). This is in line with findings that major depressive disorder in adults is associated with lower reflective functioning in general (Fischer-Kern et al., 2013) and also with lower reflective functioning specifically regarding experiences of rejection and loss (Staun, Kessler, Buchheim, Kächele, & Taubner, 2010). Vulnerability to depression has been linked to insecure attachment, especially to preoccupied and avoidant attachment (Bifulco, Moran, Ball, & Bernazzani, 2002), and the symptoms of depression may both be caused by impaired mentalizing and in turn lead to further disruptions in mentalizing (Luyten, Fonagy, Lemma, & Target, 2012). Haslam-Hopwood et al. (2006) suggested that those with depression are likely to lack the incentive to mentalize others ("why bother?"). They noted that the self-absorption and social isolation that can be features of depression may lead those with the disorder to be out of touch with the mental states of others, or indeed to be unaware of the impact of the self on relationships. Moreover, distortions in mentalizing are likely to underlie the negative cognitive bias that is a well-known feature of depression—not so much failing to read the intentions of others, but rather misreading those intentions (e.g., "He's probably just playing with me to be kind; he doesn't really want to be here.").

Childhood externalizing difficulties have also been shown to be linked to low child mentalizing as well as parental mentalizing (Ensink, Bégin, Normandin, & Fonagy, 2016; Ensink, Bégin, Normandin, Godbout, & Fonagy, 2016). Child conduct disorders, as well as oppositional defiant disorders, have been shown to be associated with lower maternal mindedness, that is, where mothers use fewer mental-state comments when interacting with young children (Centifanti, Meins, & Fernyhough, 2016; Meins, Centifanti, Fernyhough, & Fishburn, 2013). Furthermore, disorganized attachment has also been shown to be an important risk factor for later oppositional controlling behaviors (Roskam et al., 2011). In terms of the mechanisms linking low parental mentalizing and child externalizing behaviors, the parent's focus on behavior rather than trying to look past the behavior to what this may say about what the child is feeling and struggling with, may contribute to dysregulation. Furthermore, insensitive reactions to a child's oppositional and externalizing behaviors, and the parent's own difficulties in regulating infant distress, likely contribute to escalating conflict and oppositional behaviors. This may then contribute to the child becoming increasingly dysregulated and disorganized, in turn reducing the parent's capacity to mentalize.

For children who present with externalizing difficulties, interpersonal difficulties are a key feature, and Dodge, Laird, Lochman, Zelli, and the Conduct Problems Prevention Research Group (2002) showed that these children often demonstrate a range of social-cognitive deficits, including in emotional understanding and theory of mind (Hughes & Ensor, 2008). They also have a tendency to attribute hostile intentions to others when a situation is ambiguous, a form of distorted mentalizing that Sharp and Venta (2012) described as a "theory of nasty minds." Sharp, Ha, and Fonagy (2011) showed that children with behavioral problems show anomalies in their trust behavior, especially in situations in which the emotional intensity of the situation was heightened. Compared with other children, they tend to read malevolence in the intentions of others, creating a kind of epistemic hypervigilance that might prevent them from being able to make use of others in a social learning context.

In the case of callous and unemotional traits, when children may have the cognitive knowledge that someone else is suffering or in pain but lack an empathic response, it is much more difficult to determine the nature of the relationship between such problems and mentalization. There is evidence that lacking empathy and showing callousness may be partly genetic (with some overlap with some difficulties on the autistic spectrum) and that this may underlie psychopathic tendencies. On the other hand, social experiences have also been shown to activate the development of empathy, so that young children who lack empathy need to be given the chance to develop it through therapeutic relationship interventions designed to encourage perspective taking and identification and that challenge and make them aware of and question their unempathic responses. For some children with the most severe forms of externalizing problems, including those who bully or demonstrate psychopathic tendencies, there is some evidence that they are actually quite adept at reading the minds of others but that they use this skill to manipulate and control and have difficulty feeling positively connected and attached to others. Allen, Fonagy, and Bateman (2008) described this as *pseudo-mentalizing*, meaning there is a lack of true curiosity, empathy, or respect for the minds of others, even when someone may appear to be skilled at reading the mind of others. Such pseudo-mentalizing may develop in response to environments characterized by harsh and inconsistent discipline (Sharp & Venta, 2012). While this way of relating to others may be difficult to change in adults, the verdict is still out in terms of whether youngsters with such tendencies can be helped, if not necessarily to change, to become more aware of their difficulties in these areas so as to protect their close relationships.

Last but by no means least, recent research on adolescents with features of *BPD* has suggested that *hypermentalizing*—that is, overinterpretative mental state reasoning—is highly characteristic of individuals with BPD, many of whom have experienced trauma and abuse in their early lives (Sharp et al., 2011). These young people tend to overinterpret social signs and make overly complex inferences based on social cues. For example, a young girl might respond to a peer offering her support by imagining that the peer is doing this to earn her trust so that she can take advantage of her. Sharp and Venta (2012) concluded that such hypermentalization in young people with BPD is "not the result of mind-blindness; rather, individuals with BPD tend to struggle with the integration and differentiation of mental states, especially under conditions of high emotional arousal" (p. 40).

CONCLUSION

As we hope this chapter has made clear, breakdowns in mentalizing play a role in numerous childhood difficulties and are also an important concern for parents, who play a significant role in supporting their children's emotional and psychological development. Although not all problems that lead parents and caregivers to seek psychological help for their children are necessarily caused by breakdowns or deficits in mentalization, it seems likely that developing mentalizing capacities—in both parents and children—may help them develop the internal resources to face such difficulties more effectively. Moreover, recognizing the ways in which mentalizing may go awry, as well as the nonmentalizing patterns that we are likely to see in clinical settings is important to clinicians as we begin the challenging work of providing effective therapeutic interventions.

II

DESCRIPTION OF THE THERAPEUTIC APPROACH

3

THE STRUCTURE AND AIMS
OF TIME-LIMITED MBT–C

As the chapters in Part I of this book have set out, when children fail to develop a sufficient capacity to mentalize, they are deprived of a valuable tool—a skill that is at the heart of the capacity to self-regulate and to manage an increasingly complex, interpersonal world. Entering middle childhood, the capacity to mentalize is for interpersonal relations what a healthy diet might be for physical health: It creates resilience in the face of hardship and offers internal resources in the face of a demanding external world.

For many clinicians working in public and private health care settings, it is essential to be able to offer relatively brief interventions that can be of benefit to children and families. Although we have an increasing number of evidence-based treatments in child mental health, most are designed to treat specific diagnoses or symptoms, often with a behavioral focus on offering children and their parents "strategies" to manage their problems more effectively. Although such strategies can be helpful, many of those working

http://dx.doi.org/10.1037/0000028-004
Mentalization-Based Treatment for Children: A Time-Limited Approach, by N. Midgley, K. Ensink, K. Lindqvist, N. Malberg, and N. Muller

in child mental health have probably had experience of working with parents and children who struggle to use such strategies, often because they do not have the necessary affect-regulation skills or epistemic trust. By focusing on a core capacity that may promote resilience in children with a variety of presenting problems, mentalization-based treatment for children (MBT–C) aims to be a generic therapy that can be adapted to the particular needs of children in middle childhood—roughly between the ages of 5 and 12. When discussing the concept of resilience, Fonagy, Luyten, Allison, and Campbell (2016) wrote,

> Studies suggest that the ability to continue to mentalize even under considerable stress leads to so-called broaden and build (Fredrickson, 2001) cycles of attachment security, which reinforce feelings of secure attachment, personal agency, and affect regulation ("build") and lead one to be pulled into different and more adaptive environments ("broaden"). (p. 792)

These are precisely the aims of MBT–C, a time-limited, focused intervention that draws on fundamental psychodynamic principles but that can be easily integrated and used alongside various psychosocial treatments. The overall aim of MBT–C is to promote mentalizing and resilience in such a way that a developmental process is put back on track, and the family and child feel better equipped both to tackle the problems that first brought them to therapy and to learn how to make better use of supportive relationships. In doing this, MBT–C aims to increase the child's capacity for emotional regulation and to support parents to best meet the emotional needs of their children.

Working with parents alongside the time-limited therapy with the child is seen as an essential element of MBT–C, not only in the short-term but also to give the best possibility that the parents will continue to support the child's development after the therapy has ended. For some children, a time-limited MBT treatment may be all that is needed; for others, it can be seen as a starting point to develop reflective and regulatory capacities, which may need additional, longer term support or therapy to ensure that development stays on track. As in many other time-limited therapies, we do not always expect an entire process of change to take place within therapy, but rather, we aim to start a change process that can continue after therapy has ended (Allen, O'Malley, Freeman, & Bateman, 2012).

In this chapter, we begin by presenting our views on which children may benefit most from time-limited MBT–C. We then describe the overarching aims of this therapy, both in direct work with children and in parallel work with parents. Next, we provide an overview of the main treatment phases in MBT–C, each of which is described in more detail in subsequent chapters.

WHICH CHILDREN MIGHT BENEFIT
FROM TIME-LIMITED MBT–C?

Time-limited MBT–C was developed for children between the ages of 5 and 12 years who present with a range of emotional and behavioral difficulties. Because this approach is still in the early stages of its development, there is as yet no systematic evidence to identify which children are most likely to benefit. So although the guidance in this chapter must be provisional, it is based on practice-based evidence, having been tested in various clinical settings. What we hope to offer are some clinically useful guidelines on when to offer time-limited MBT–C, but as with all guidelines, these will need to form the basis for more systematic research and evaluation, which will in turn inform our ongoing understanding of "what works, for whom."

Because of its focus on promoting a core developmental process, MBT–C has not been developed specifically for treating one type of clinical presentation. In Chapter 2, we outlined what the empirical research suggests about the role of mentalizing in different childhood disorders. Informed by that research, as well as our own clinical experience, we suggest that MBT–C may be suitable primarily for children presenting with affective or anxiety disorders, mild or moderate behavior problems, as well as those with adjustment reactions or who need help dealing with a particular life challenge, such as parental divorce or bereavement. In some cases, as we discuss later, time-limited MBT–C may also be recommended for those who have experienced trauma and attachment difficulties. With regard to attachment disorders, our experience is that these children can benefit from this model, and in the case studies that we use throughout this book, we have tried to show how this may be the case. However, caution is needed when recommending time-limited MBT–C for children with more severe externalizing disorders, as well as severe attachment disorders or neurodevelopmental disorders, and in all cases, careful consideration of the child's particular circumstances should inform any treatment recommendation.

Although nonbehavioral therapies generally report less successful outcomes for children with externalizing problems, there is a particular reason why we do not rule out time-limited MBT–C as a treatment for all children with behavioral problems. In many cases of externalizing and aggressive children, parents as well as clinicians often focus on the "noisy" symptoms, while missing co-occurring internalizing symptoms, such as anxiety, depression, or low self-confidence (Goodman, Stroh, & Valdez, 2012). Many children with conduct problems have received little help in understanding and integrating aspects of their temperament such as impulsivity, aggression, competitiveness, or dominance and may benefit enormously from the opportunity to think about this with someone who is curious rather than judgmental. In such cases, a therapist can help the child develop self-awareness and potentially explore more adaptive ways of integrating these aspects of their temperament or personality to help facilitate self-esteem and affect regulation.

We are more hesitant to make claims that this treatment can be effective if a lack of empathy underlies aggressive behaviors (e.g., children with callous/unemotional traits) or if there is a sadistic quality to the aggression. However, it may be worthwhile to attempt to stimulate the development of empathy and an awareness of the negative effects aggression has on others, given that there is much to gain and little to lose by intervening.

For children with experiences of trauma or loss, the therapist needs to assess the extent and severity of the trauma to establish whether a time-limited model is suitable or sufficient. Children who have suffered from severe maltreatment, trauma, or emotional neglect often evoke so much worry in the adults around them that it can be difficult to look past their own reactions to the traumatic events and concerns about their possible impact to see the child. A treatment that focuses on the child's mind and experiences in a relational context may well be of benefit, although there should be no illusion that short-term work can undo the effects of severe and enduring trauma. Nonetheless, for some chronically traumatized children, the time limitation may help them to commit to the process because therapy can appear less threatening.

Likewise, for children with multiple experiences of separation and disruption, there may be reason to reflect on whether a time-limited model is appropriate. For most children, the separation from the therapist after a time-limited intervention is an opportunity to work through a well-prepared ending, as we discuss more fully in Chapter 8. However, for some children who have had multiple rejections (e.g., those who have had multiple moves among different foster families), ending and separating so soon after establishing a bond, perhaps for the first time, may not be therapeutic. With these children, we recommend that the therapist make a careful clinical evaluation and embark cautiously on time-limited psychotherapy, with the notion that more extended treatment may be needed.

Neurodevelopmental disorders, such as autistic spectrum disorder (ASD) and pervasive developmental disorder (PDD), are not absolute counterindications for time-limited MBT–C. On the contrary, children with these difficulties can benefit from this way of working, possibly with some modifications. However, we want to underscore that these conditions are not the target for treatment but that children should not be excluded from treatment exclusively on the basis of having these diagnoses. Children may be able to benefit from time-limited MBT–C despite these difficulties and in fact may be particularly in need of help with developing mentalizing skills around specific key issues or difficulties, while accepting that their abilities are different. For example, children with ASD may need help exploring their feelings of exclusion and in considering what they may realistically be able to expect in the future, what they have to accept and what they may be able to change, and to develop ways that they may address certain social deficits. In setting goals, being realistic about what to expect from therapy is even more essential for children in whom there are many core issues that cannot be expected to be resolved with time-limited psychotherapy.

As the preceding paragraphs make clear, making treatment recommendations based purely on psychiatric diagnosis is of limited value. We suggest instead that MBT–C is suitable for children with a wide range of clinical difficulties and that MBT–C is flexible so that therapists can adjust how they will work to ensure the process is appropriate for particular children, considering their level of functioning and the limits of their capacities. In light of what we have said in the first two chapters about the importance of epistemic trust, one factor to consider when thinking about suitability for MBT–C is the nature and quality of the child's capacity to consider new knowledge from another person as trustworthy, generalizable, and relevant to the self (Fonagy & Allison, 2014). When there is a fundamental capacity for epistemic trust, the child and parents are open to the therapist and open to learn. This is most often found in children with specific or temporary mentalizing breakdowns who have perhaps faced situations that have challenged their functioning, such as parental separation or a significant loss.

When a child or their parents (or both) have a greater degree of epistemic distrust, more time may be needed to build a relationship to the therapist(s), but the argument for offering a more mentalization-focused intervention is stronger because the focus of the work explicitly focuses on addressing what may stop the child or parent from being able to learn from others. However, the process of generalizing what is learned in therapy may take longer because of the mistrust that can only gradually change into trusting oneself and others. As described in the previous chapter, this is more often the case for children with insecure attachments, where helping to address the child's epistemic vigilance and suspicion toward others may be a core part of the therapeutic work. When parents share such suspicion, it is especially important to engage them meaningfully in the work.

Children who have experienced chronic trauma, such as neglect or abuse, or who have disorganized patterns of attachment, often show epistemic hypervigilance. When presenting for services, these children may display a combination of internalizing and externalizing problems. Rigidity and instability are common features, and there is a high risk of emerging personality problems. For many of these children, a short period of time-limited MBT–C will not be enough. However, this is not to say that offering open-ended, long-term work is necessarily the better option. Haugvik and Johns (2006, 2008) have pointed out that offering a focused, time-limited therapy can often help families with more complex problems engage in therapy. Offering an initial period of time-limited work can be extremely helpful, but it is also important to be realistic and modest about the aims of the work. So, too, when the parents themselves have severe psychiatric difficulties, careful thought needs to be given to whether a time-limited MBT–C approach is appropriate.

OVERARCHING AIMS OF TIME-LIMITED MBT–C

Although the clinical presentations of children entering time-limited MBT–C may vary, there are certain aims of the work that are likely to be common. The general aim of MBT–C is to help develop and enhance mentalizing processes in the child but also in the parents, which will in turn help the child to become aware of and regulate emotions and/or develop explicit mentalizing skills that can help them manage key difficulties. These key difficulties can be addressing trauma, parental mental illness or other family and life difficulties, or developing better mentalizing about aspects of self, such as temperament or specific emotional difficulties and concerns. Related to this is helping the child create a narrative and develop a more coherent sense of self, which can lead to a more positive self-image. When a child has a capacity to mentalize about their reactions and those of others, this should facilitate emotion regulation and contribute to a feeling of self-agency.

A central aim of the individual work with the child is to develop the capacity to recognize, endure, and regulate emotions. This capacity is enormously helpful in becoming more attuned to others and understanding complex social situations, as well as experiencing self-control, a sense of self, and agency. Children brought to therapy may be either underregulated or overregulated, meaning that feelings can be experienced and expressed too little or too much. It is not unusual for children to underregulate certain affects and overregulate others. For example, a child may overregulate anxiety about separation, appearing to be dismissive of attachment needs, yet underregulate when it comes to his capacity to control aggression. The aim in therapy is to help the child develop the capacity to identify, regulate, and express emotions in age-appropriate ways.

A metaphor that might illustrate this and can be helpful for parents is to talk about affect regulation as a form of *volume control*. When children have limited capacities for affect regulation, we may think of it in terms of them needing to learn to use their volume control more effectively: Sometimes the volume is too low, so that their feelings can't be heard by themselves and those around them; sometimes the volume is too high, so that their feelings take over, and it is impossible to hear anything else, such as their own thoughts. To use their volume control effectively, they first need to recognize that there is something there that they may need to modulate. The second step is finding the volume control, and the third step is actually using the volume control and regulating and modulating.

For children who have experienced breakdowns in mentalization due to trauma, loss, or other specific triggering situations or events, an additional aim can be to *create a coherent narrative* about the event, as well as to explore related thoughts, feelings, and experiences. A crucial element of this is mentalizing the affect (Jurist, 2005), which is at the heart of regulating emotions. This means reflecting on emotions linked to traumatic events or losses and accepting the existence of feelings without being overwhelmed by them. The aim is not to create insight into the trauma but to learn and understand in the here-and-now how to endure and regulate the emotions associated with the traumatic event.

Another aim common to most MBT–C work is to strengthen and deepen the child's ability to *form and maintain relationships*. Related to this is to work with affective interaction—to be able to regulate and express emotions in relationships. This can also entail seeking comfort and care from attachment figures when in distress.

Alongside the direct work with the child, the fundamental aim of the work with parents is to strengthen their *parental reflective functioning* (Slade, 2005) and capacity for assuming a reflective stance as parents (Ensink, Leroux, Normandin, Biberdzic, & Fonagy, in press). This includes helping them to develop a capacity to think about the child's psychological experience and focus on the child's mind and to see their child as a separate person with his or her own thoughts and feelings, with a sense that being curious about their child's mind can help parents to give meaning to behaviors. A secondary, but nonetheless important, component is also to help parents develop the capacity to see their own affects and behavior from the perspective of their child because this may have an impact on their parenting in important ways. When parents can explicitly mentalize about themselves and their child, they may respond to the child's needs and emotions in more flexible and attuned ways.

Inevitably, parents of children referred for therapy, like all of us, will have their own mentalizing difficulties, whether temporary or more pervasive. Helping parents reflect on how their emotions affect their behavior toward the child, and in turn influence their child's emotions, is thus an important part of the work. Developing, for example, empathic awareness of when their own anger may be overwhelming, disorganizing, and scary (for the child but also perhaps for themselves), or how fear and anxiety makes them withdraw or become intrusive and controlling, may have crucial implications for their capacity to limit potentially harmful interactions with their children. Parents who experienced neglect or abuse in their own childhood may need extra help to address real or imagined concerns around intergenerational patterns that may affect their parenting.

In light of recent work related to the concept of epistemic trust, it is possible to think about the general aims of MBT–C in an additional way. Fonagy and Allison (2014), in writing about their work with adults who have personality disorders, suggested that learning to mentalize in treatment is not, in itself, a sufficient therapeutic aim. Instead, they argued that mentalizing in therapy is only of value as a way of establishing epistemic trust: "The very experience of having our subjectivity understood—of being mentalized—is a necessary trigger for us to be able to receive and learn from the social knowledge that has the potential to change our perception of ourselves and our social world" (p. 372).

In light of these ideas, Fonagy and Allison (2014) described the key processes that they consider to underlie all meaningful therapeutic change:

- First is the development of a therapeutic context in which patients feel understood, which allows them to reduce their sense of epistemic mistrust or hypervigilance.
- Second is the reemergence of patients' capacity to mentalize, as they *find themselves in the mind of the therapist*, leading to a greater sense of self-coherence and agency.
- Third is recovery of a "capacity for social information exchange" (p. 377), which allows the patient to discover new ways of learning from, and about, others beyond the therapy context.

Although these authors were writing about therapeutic work with adults with personality disorders, we find these ideas helpful when thinking about time-limited MBT with children as well. This is partly because they have made explicit why work with parents is such a crucial part of the model. Fonagy and Campbell (2015) noted that when speaking about work with adult patients,

> reopening epistemic trust in a therapeutic context is merely one part of a process of social learning . . . that needs to be supported in the patient's wider social environment for there to be any chance of sustained or meaningful change. (p. 243)

If this is true of adults, it is even more the case in work with children, whose ongoing dependence on their caregivers makes it essential to help create the kind of context(s) in which the child is able to continue to benefit from the changes that, we hope, can begin in therapy.

Although time-limited therapy may not be sufficient to fully restore a sense of epistemic trust, it is possible to address or make children aware that certain early experiences may have affected their trust in others and in life and thus begin a process of *epistemic unfreezing*. It may be helpful for children to feel how lack of trust may manifest in their interpersonal relationships with peers and family, for example, always wanting to lead and being afraid to let go, which might make them come across as domineering to other children. An important experience when a child lacks this sense of epistemic trust is starting the process of daring to trust others. This can happen when another person (initially the therapist but also the other adults or caregivers in the child's life) reacts with respect and curiosity toward them. Thus, the process of restoring epistemic trust and social learning can be started in a time-limited therapy.

STRUCTURE AND FRAME OF TIME-LIMITED MBT–C

To be able to explore, we need a secure base that we know we can return to if necessary. In therapeutic work with children and families, we strive to help parents become the secure base from which their child can explore the world, and we invite children to develop a curiosity about their own mind and the minds of others. To feel safe in undertaking this process, children require a secure external world where they feel in control (Blake, 2008). Many children and parents with mentalizing problems do not experience the outer, or the inner, world as safe enough for this exploration to take place. In MBT–C, the therapist strives to create an atmosphere of safety. A clear, transparent, and predictable therapeutic frame is one important factor in achieving that.

The specific practicalities of the frame include a time limitation with a predefined number of sessions, a calendar, a focus formulation, and parallel work with the parent(s). The standard duration of time-limited MBT–C is 12 weekly sessions. We aim to not be overly prescriptive because the practicalities of the treatment can be organized in several ways, depending on clinical setting and the severity of the problems the child and parents describe. What is important is that the therapeutic contract is clear and coherent from the beginning—for the parents as well as the child. This creates a sense of safety and collaboration and avoids a scenario in which the therapist makes decisions without the family's knowledge or input. This transparency is part of the mentalizing stance, described more fully in Chapter 4, and contributes to a sense of shared ownership of the therapeutic process.

The notion of "phases" in therapy is to some degree artificial, given that the underlying aims and techniques of the work continue from the beginning to the end of therapy. Nevertheless, part of the structure of time-limited MBT–C is a predictable shape to the treatment, which can be thought of in terms of key phases, each with its own particular tasks (see Exhibit 3.1).

EXHIBIT 3.1
The Phases of Treatment in MBT–C

Assessment Phase (3–4 Meetings)
Assessment meetings are held with family, child, and parents.
The assessment phase is reviewed, including offering feedback on the assessment, making decisions about continuing with MBT–C, and sharing and discussing the focus formulation and goals.

- **Sessions 1–3: Initial Phase**
  With the child: Introduce the calendar and therapy box to the child, focus on engaging the child in treatment, and explore whether the child can play around the focus formulation.
  With the parent(s): Focus on engaging parent(s) in treatment, work with the parents around the focus formulation, and support reflective parenting.
- **Sessions 4–8: Middle Phase**
  The focus of work with parents and the child is on stimulating and developing mentalizing capacity in relation to the focus formulation and the issues that brought the child to therapy.
- **After Session 8: Review Meeting**
  In a joint meeting with both therapists (if there are two) and parents, the progress of therapy is reviewed to make a decision about whether to move toward ending, offer additional sessions, or recommend alternative approaches.
- **Sessions 9–12: Ending Phase**
  When therapy is due to end, the focus is on preparing for the ending and exploring how best to maintain gains beyond the end of therapy.
  If therapy will continue, work with the parents and child will be ongoing.
- **3–12 Months After Ending: Checking-In or Booster Sessions**

Note. MBT–C = mentalization-based treatment for children.

Assessment Phase (3–4 Meetings Before Beginning MBT–C)

All therapeutic work with children and their families should be based on a thorough assessment leading to some provisional understanding of the presenting problem(s), as well as a formulation of how those problems may be linked to the proposed intervention. Depending on the context in which therapists work, there may already be particular approaches to how an assessment is conducted; however, in Chapter 5, we set out a model of assessment that focuses on developing a *mentalizing profile* of the child and family. The aim of such an assessment is to explore whether and how mentalizing difficulties may be linked to the child's presenting problems and whether a mentalization-focused intervention is likely to be of help.

The model of assessment set out in this book shows how the MBT–C therapist can assess the capacity to mentalize in both children and parents, offer feedback on the assessment, and make decisions with families about whether to continue with MBT–C. If work is to proceed, a focus statement is formulated, and the child, parents, and therapist will agree on a set of goals for the treatment.

Sessions 1–3: Initial Phase of MBT–C

Although it can be thought of as a separate phase of treatment, much of what is done during the first few sessions in MBT–C builds on the work already done in the assessment phase (Chapter 5) and makes use of techniques that are also part of the ongoing sessions with the child (Chapter 6). With children, the primary aim of this initial phase is to establish a therapeutic alliance, primarily through means of empathic attunement and genuine engagement with and curiosity about the child's world. As is discussed more fully in Chapter 6, play is central to this process of engagement and is a marvelous way to socialize the child to the way that therapy works. This will include introducing the calendar and the therapy box to the child and exploring whether the child can play around the focus formulation. With parent(s), engagement and establishing a therapeutic alliance are also paramount as the parent therapist begins to support *reflective parenting* (Chapter 7). Empathic attunement with the parent's experience, even when the therapist may have different views on how a parent is responding to their child, is key at this stage.

Sessions 4–8: The Middle Phase

The middle phase of the work (approximately sessions 4–8) is where the core work on developing the child's mentalizing capacity takes place, drawing on numerous therapeutic techniques and in relation to the focus formulation (see Chapter 6). Meanwhile, the sessions with parents can increasingly focus on promoting the various elements of reflective parenting. In the work with both parents and children, if affects can be regulated in a way that makes explicit mentalizing possible, then empathic attunement can increasingly be complemented by a focus on promoting perspective-taking and seeing things from others' points of view. In some cases, the focus will be more on promoting the underdeveloped capacity for mentalizing or paying attention to the situations in which explicit mentalizing breaks down.

Review Meeting

After the first eight sessions, a *review meeting* is offered with the child and parents in which the initial focus and treatment goals are reviewed and it is decided whether the initial block of sessions seems sufficient or whether work needs to continue or may be approaching an ending (see Chapter 8). When it is felt that the therapeutic work will need to go on for longer than the initial block of sessions, it is still possible to work in a time-limited way using an *open-ticket-model*. In this case, another block of 12 sessions can be offered, up to a maximum of 36 (three 12-session blocks) sessions. This flexibility facilitates the time-limited approach for children with more complex disorders, such as those who have experienced trauma or have attachment disorders. However, we do not necessarily believe that more complex difficulties always benefit from longer (or open-ended) therapies. Our experience is that working with a time limitation and a focus can be helpful but that children with more complex problems often need more than one block of 12 sessions.

Sessions 9–12: Ending Phase

When therapy is due to end, the focus is on preparing for the ending and exploring how best to maintain the gains that have been made beyond the end of treatment. As is described more fully in Chapter 8, the time-limited nature of MBT–C means that endings are kept actively in mind throughout the work, and the use of a calendar helps children understand how many sessions they have had, and how many are left. Because one of the aims of MBT–C is to ensure that the child and parents end the therapy with a better capacity to make use of other relationships outside therapy, a particular focus of the ending phase is on translating what has been learned in therapy to other supportive relationships.

Checking-In or Booster Sessions

At whatever point the time-limited therapy ends, the MBT–C model includes a checking-in or *booster session*, which is arranged anywhere between 3 and 12 months after the completion of treatment. The timing of this meeting and how it should be planned are discussed in Chapter 8.

THE PHYSICAL SETTING FOR THERAPY

When thinking about an optimal setting for therapy with children, there are no clear prescriptions. We recommend that the therapy be conducted in the same room for all sessions and that this room not change too much between sessions. Sometimes, however, the location may need to be changed when there is reason to believe that the child needs a specific context. For example, in some settings, there may be an outdoor space that is available to the therapist or a gym where the child is able to engage in more physical activities. Moving the therapy to such a setting at certain points can be helpful for children with attention-regulation problems, such as those who are hyperactive or aggressive or who are quickly overwhelmed by incentives from the outside and lack regulation capacities.

A child's therapy room does not necessarily need to contain a lot of toys or play material. On the contrary, children with regulation difficulties may become overwhelmed in rooms with too many of such items to choose from. When the arousal level is too high, children will not be able to play or pay attention to what they are experiencing. Likewise, some children may feel safer in a smaller room, whereas others may need the space of a bigger room so as not to feel restricted. Ideally, the room needs to have at least some floor space large enough for the child to move around and play more physical games, such as looping a ball into a basket, playing mini-hockey, or simply throwing and catching a ball. Having some personal things in the room may be helpful for some children because they might recognize aspects of the therapist in the way the room is styled and because this can create a less institutional atmosphere (Slijper, 2008). At the same time, some children may feel anxious or have feelings of rivalry toward other children when a room is too personal.

When selecting playroom materials, the therapist aims to create the optimal space for children to play and express themselves. It is recommended that some sensory or sensopathic play materials that stimulate or awaken the senses be available. As Stern (1992, 2004) has pointed out, such materials are often important for children with attention- and affect-regulation problems. These can include a sand tray or kinetic sand, clay, finger paint, water, bubbles, or different sizes and types of balls. To stimulate fantasy and role-play, dolls, animal figures, cars, bricks, and dress-up clothes are often used, and it is valuable to have dolls with a variety of skin tones and of different genders and ages. It is also a good idea to have a few games as part of the playroom material. Almost all therapists have some art supplies, and some therapists also have other creative materials, such as musical instruments. Of course, as therapists, we do not always have much control over what kind of space is available or what materials are provided, but even so, it can be helpful to think with the child and parents about how the space may be experienced and how it may affect the child's behavior in sessions. The aim is for the child to feel invited and at ease to play following their impulses (within certain limits) and to express themselves freely.

TIME AS A FRAMEWORK FOR THERAPY

The British child psychotherapist Monica Lanyado (2012) wrote that

child psychotherapy is about holding and letting go. The balance between holding and letting go is an important issue in life and is a reciprocal process. Just as parents have to learn how and when to let go of the child and when to hold the child in mind more, so the child also needs to learn when it is safe to let go of the parents as well as when to seek the parents' presence, internally and externally. (p. 117)

The aspect of time is addressed throughout therapy, and its importance is emphasized by the time limitation, supported by the use of a calendar, described in more detail shortly. Time limitation can be a motivational factor to work with the most urgent issues and reminds us that the family will need to have the capacity to address difficulties for themselves in the near future. Every therapeutic intervention in MBT–C has as its ultimate aim to encourage and increase the ability to mentalize in a way that can help parents and children manage their difficulties more constructively once the treatment is over. In this way, the ending is built into the process from the very beginning of therapy (see also Chapter 9).

Being transparent about the time limitation and the number of sessions remaining also gives the child an opportunity to prepare for and work through the separation that comes with the end of therapy. Many children in therapy have experienced multiple separations in their lives, but they may not always have had the time to prepare and work through them, making this a new experience in which feelings about endings can be addressed together with the therapist. Because MBT–C is process focused, the time frame can also serve as a port of entry in terms of activating relational dynamics. For example, when a child (or indeed a parent) complains, "You don't give me enough time!" this can be used to explore triggers of nonmentalizing moments or may reflect issues of fairness for some children and families that can be helpfully explored.

Inspired by developmentally directed time-limited psychotherapy for children (Haugvik & Johns, 2006; Røed Hansen, 2012), one of the ways in which the MBT–C therapist actively works with the time limitation is by using a calendar. The aim of the calendar is to stimulate a sense of ownership of the therapy in the child, to encourage a reflective stance, and to help the child gain a sense of the time-limited nature of the work (Gydal & Knudtzon, 2002).

Calendars can look different but should always consist of a (preferably large) paper marked with as many rectangles or circles as there are sessions. The therapist introduces the calendar during the first session. As part of establishing the framework of the therapy, the therapist tells the child that at the end of each session, they will draw something in the calendar and that this is a way for them to keep track of the sessions and reflect together on what has happened that day. A good idea may be to let the child number the spaces in the calendar to establish it as a way to give some sense of the length of the therapy from the beginning. The child can also decorate the back of the calendar to make it more personal and thereby enhance the sense that it belongs to them.

When there is approximately 5 to 10 minutes remaining in a session, the therapist asks the child to draw something on the calendar. The main "rule" for this is that anything the child chooses to draw is OK. The calendar belongs to the child, and they can decide what to draw on it. There may be times when the therapist feels an urge to help the child by suggesting certain things to draw or even helping the child draw, but unless the child explicitly asks for this, the therapist should refrain. Sometimes, however, the therapist needs to take responsibility for the calendar—for example, not letting the child tear it apart, paint all over the different spaces, or otherwise ruin it.

As mentioned earlier in the chapter, one aim of MBT–C is to help the child create a coherent narrative. Using a calendar, the child and the therapist create their own story—a narrative about the therapeutic process can be created and visualized together. The calendar can also be a powerful tool for addressing the ending of the therapy and the forthcoming separation. By looking at the calendar together, the child and the therapist can keep track of the number of sessions they have left and prepare for their farewell. At the end of the therapy and in the booster sessions, the calendar can be used for looking back and reviewing the work that has been done together (Røed Hansen, 2012).

FOCUS FORMULATION

Another core aspect of the therapeutic frame, also inspired by developmentally directed time-limited psychotherapy for children (Haugvik & Johns, 2006; Røed Hansen, 2012), is formulating a focus for the therapy, which should emerge out of carefully observing and listening to what the child conveys during the assessment sessions, verbally as well as nonverbally. The focus formulation should be a short phrase or a story, shared with the child and parents at the start of treatment. In a way, it can be related to Stern's (1985) concept of a *key metaphor*, representing core relational and emotional themes (Johns, 2008). One of the main aims of the focus formulation is to convey to the child that the therapy has something to offer them. Many children are brought to therapy by parents or other adults, with the children having little knowledge of why they are there or thinking they are simply there to please the adults around them (Johns, 2008). When time is limited, the task of engaging the child becomes more urgent, and the focus can be seen as an invitation to the child to engage in the therapy process. Using material from the assessment with children to formulate the focus can strengthen their sense of agency in the therapy—something they have contributed to the encounter becomes a focus for the treatment.

Another aim with the focus formulation is to stimulate mentalizing by directing the parents' attention to central experiences, thoughts, and feelings in the child—keeping the child's mind in mind and, at the same time, stimulating the child's self-reflection around their own inner states. The therapist's formulation becomes a model for keeping someone else's mind in mind. The focus creates joint attention toward what the child presents as central experiences, thoughts, and feelings. It shows that the therapist has taken in something from the parents and child and invites a meaning-creating dialogue around the problems that brought the child to therapy. The process of formulating a focus is presented more fully in Chapter 5.

ONE THERAPIST OR TWO?

Work with parents or caregivers (and, where needed, with the wider network around the child) is considered a key component of time-limited MBT–C. The basic model is that two therapists work together, one with the child and one with the parents. Ideally, the sessions are scheduled at the same time. This gives parents and child their own space, but they still come together to the clinic, creating a sense that this is something they are doing together as a joint family effort. It is also helpful practically because it means that parents do not need to make separate visits for their own meetings. The two therapists work as a team, helping each other to keep their mentalizing "online." The collaboration between the therapists can serve as a model for the family of how to mentalize together. It can also decrease concerns regarding confidentiality for the children, especially older ones, who may have concerns that what they talk about in their sessions will be shared with the parents.

In some cases, of course, there may be practical or therapeutic reasons for working with only one therapist. First and foremost, in many private practices or clinics, therapists lack opportunities to work in pairs. But even when this is an option, there may be some situations in which one therapist is preferable. Some parents find it difficult to trust their child to anyone whom they do not know and can be more supportive of the child's therapy if they have some direct access to their child's therapist. For children to be able to use the therapeutic space and to trust the therapist, they need to feel that their parents agree they are allowed to do so. When this is not possible, loyalty conflicts may arise. Although these can create opportunities to explore mental states, such conflicts can also threaten the work and obstruct the therapeutic process. In these cases, it may help the parents if they feel that they know and have a trusting relationship with the person who is working with their child. Furthermore, in families in which there are very different views of the child or the presenting problems, intense conflicts, or significant blaming, having the same therapist may become a uniting factor. A therapist who works directly with the child can sometimes bring the child to life in their meeting with the parents in a way that is not as easy for a separate parent therapist, who inevitably focuses to a much greater extent on the child in the parent's mind.

INTRODUCING THE CASES

In the remaining chapters of this book, we use vignettes from six cases to illustrate the model of time-limited MBT with children. As outlined in the Introduction, these are composite cases that draw on our clinical experience but do not describe actual children or families with whom we have worked. We have selected these cases because we think they represent the diversity of children who might be seen in time-limited MBT–C, both in terms of their ages and the presenting problems that brought them to therapy. The children demonstrate a range of attachment strategies (some more avoidant, others more preoccupied or disorganized) and capacities for mentalizing. They are also varied in the nature of their family contexts and the capacity of their carers to mentalize the child.

Other than the chapter on assessment, where we follow one particular child (John) through the entire process, the vignettes from different children are combined in each chapter. To help the reader hold each of the children in mind, an image of that child (based on photos of child actors) are included alongside each vignette.

Anne, Age 6 Years

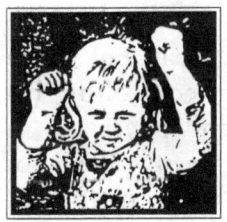 Anne was referred to therapy because of temper tantrums, oppositional behavior, and separation anxiety. She is an only child, and her parents divorced when she was 2 years old; she now lives with her mother, Mrs. H. Anne's tantrums mostly happen at home, but lately her mother has started getting calls from Anne's school regarding her tendency to push and kick other children in her class when she is frustrated. When her mother is trying to drop her off at the school, Anne often clings to her mother and doesn't want her to leave. She exhibits a high level of activity and the adults around her have noticed that it seems difficult for her to relax and be calm. Mrs. H can sometimes feel so helpless that she locks herself in a room at home while Anne is left screaming downstairs.

Mohammed, Age 7 Years

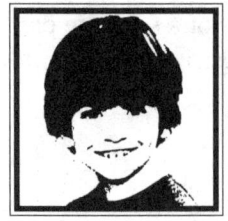 Mohammed was in a severe car accident 6 months ago and injured his leg badly. His parents are divorced, and he lives primarily with his father, Mr. D, who has a new partner. After the accident, Mohammed began having aggressive outbursts at home and school. He has always been an active and smart boy who likes getting his way, but his father says he has become especially difficult to negotiate with since the accident. He has difficulties sleeping and complains of nightmares. Mr. D describes how Mohammed used to be an "easy" and well-tempered child but lately has been highly irritable and unpredictable in his behavior.

Belinda, Age 7 Years

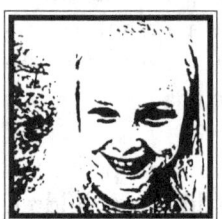 Belinda's mother contacted the clinic worrying that Belinda was often sad. Belinda lives with her mother, Mrs. C, and grandmother; she has no contact with her father or half-sister. The school reports no difficulties, but Mrs. C says there is a struggle every morning to get Belinda out of bed, dressed, and on the school bus. Belinda says that she doesn't like school, and when her mother or grandmother try to "talk her into a better mood," she can become quite cruel. Both mother and grandmother say that they feel controlled by Belinda and rather hopeless about how best to help her.

John, Age 8 Years

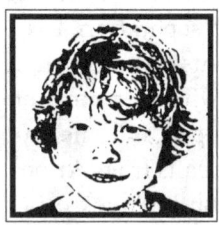 John was referred for therapy because of severe aggressive outbursts and difficulty controlling his impulses. He acts out verbally and physically at school as well as at home. His aggressive behavior makes him isolated at school, and he has no friends. John lives in a foster family with a foster mother and father and two foster sisters, having been removed from his parents at age 2. His father disappeared when he was a baby, and his mother suffers from severe, ongoing psychiatric difficulties. John sometimes visits his biological mother, who has a new partner and lives with John's biological brother. He has previously lived with two other foster families.

Liza, Age 11 Years

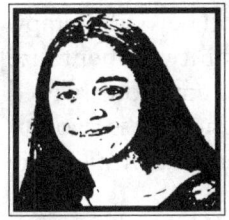

Liza has always been shy but lately has increasingly struggled with any kind of separation from her mother. She has stomach pains and headaches when going to school and calls her mother several times a day. She is withdrawn in school and has few friends there. Liza lives with her mother, father, and brother (age 15). Her brother can sometimes behave quite violently outside the home, has been involved in street crime, and frequently argues with his parents. There is a lot of conflict in the family related to her brother, and the parents describe themselves as being under considerable stress because of their son's behavior. They worry that Liza's needs have been somewhat neglected because they have had so much difficulty with her brother over the years, who is now supported by a specialist youth-offending team.

Ruth, Age 12 Years

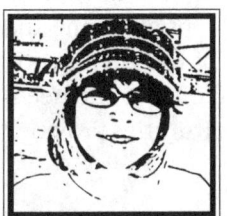

Ruth comes to therapy with her foster parents, two women with whom she has been living for the past 2 years. Ruth was born in prison, and her biological parents are both still incarcerated. During her childhood, she has lived in different foster homes. In one of the foster homes, she witnessed a sexual act between her foster siblings, which had a traumatic effect on her and led to her being moved to her current foster parents. Ruth has temper tantrums, difficulties eating, and mood swings; at times, she can be bossy and aggressive, and at other times, she can become sad and withdrawn.

CONCLUDING REMARKS

Time-limited MBT–C has been developed for use with children with various presenting problems and is not a therapy developed to treat children with only one specific diagnosis. When assessing suitability and planning the treatment, a comprehensive review of the child and family functioning is needed, one that pays attention to not only symptoms and behavior but also to the nature and severity of the mentalizing deficits, especially whether there is a global underdevelopment of mentalizing or the breakdowns in mentalizing are more specific or temporary.

The overarching aim of time-limited MBT–C is to help develop and enhance mentalizing processes, helping the child to become aware of and regulate emotions and to mentalize about difficulties that they might face. This in turn can help reduce epistemic mistrust, so that the child is better able to make use of supportive relationships, both within and beyond therapy. The aim of the parental work is to enhance the carers' ability to mentalize regarding their child's experiences, as well as parents' own emotions related to parenting and how they influence family interactions. When these two can be achieved side by side, children with a range of presenting difficulties may be meaningfully helped.

The standard model for MBT–C is 12 sessions for the child, with simultaneous sessions for the parents, but it leaves room for adaptation. The calendar and the focus statement become means for the child to develop a sense of participation, ownership, and agency in the therapeutic process and are helpful instruments for keeping track of time and creating coherency in the therapy. In time-limited MBT–C, structure and focus are seen as important therapeutic factors. Having everybody agree on the setting of the therapy from the start enhances the sense that the therapeutic endeavor is a shared one and that the therapist does not have "privileged" information or make decisions on their own. By discussing aspects of the therapeutic setting together with the family, therapists can model a reflective stance and negotiate an appropriate frame and a focus statement for therapy. Nevertheless, many aspects of the therapeutic frame, such as working with one or two therapists, can be tailored to the needs of the family, the preferences of the clinicians, and the opportunities provided in the clinical setting.

4

THE THERAPIST STANCE IN TIME-LIMITED MBT–C

Successful mentalizing is not so much the capacity to always accurately read one's own or another's inner states, but rather a way of approaching relationships that reflects an expectation that one's own thinking and feeling may be enlightened, enriched, and changed by learning about the mental states of other people. In this respect, mentalizing is as much an attitude as it is a skill, an attitude which is inquiring and respectful of other people's mental states, aware of the limits of one's knowledge of others and reflects a view that understanding the feelings of others is important for maintaining healthy and mutually rewarding relationships. (Fearon, as cited in Bevington, n.d.)

When teaching mentalization-based treatment (MBT) to therapists who are new to the approach, there is often a temptation to focus on acquiring specific techniques, as if they are the heart of any therapeutic approach. But as most people working in this field would probably agree, any specific model

http://dx.doi.org/10.1037/0000028-005
Mentalization-Based Treatment for Children: A Time-Limited Approach, by N. Midgley, K. Ensink, K. Lindqvist, N. Malberg, and N. Muller

of therapy—whether MBT, cognitive behavior therapy, psychodynamic therapy, or interpersonal therapy—is not simply a set of tools or techniques that can be "applied" when working with children and families; it also implies a stance, or way of being, that informs every aspect of the therapeutic work.

When researchers ask adults or children to look back on what it was like going to therapy, few of them say much about what kind of techniques the therapist used; they don't often comment on the quality of the cognitive reframing or whether the therapist's interpretations were accurate; instead, they tend to begin by speaking about the person of the therapist—what was she like? Was she nice? Did they feel comfortable with her? Of course, this doesn't mean that the techniques the therapist uses do not matter, but that all such techniques always take place in the context of a relationship and that therapists' "way of being" may be as important as the particular techniques that we use.

The therapist's stance in MBT is not simply in the background as the "real work" of therapy is conducted; it is at the core of what MBT is and how it works. It is for this reason that we introduce it here, before presenting the specific details of the MBT for children (MBT–C) model itself. The stance is crucial because it is both an aim of MBT–C insofar as we are trying to help the families we work with to develop the capacity to mentalize but also the means through which we can achieve this aim by trying to model this stance ourselves. Exhibit 4.1 presents the key elements of the therapeutic stance in MBT–C.

This chapter therefore sets out the key components of this mentalizing stance, including the importance of curiosity, humor, and an interest in exploring the perspective of others. Most important, we describe the ways in which the therapist's own mentalizing capacity can break down and the importance of identifying these moments and using them for therapeutic ends. We end by making some comments about the role of supervision in supporting the therapist's mentalizing stance and describe an approach to supervision that focuses explicitly on helping therapists to maintain their own capacity to mentalize.

EXHIBIT 4.1
Key Elements of the Therapeutic Stance in MBT–C

- The therapeutic presence of the MBT–C therapist (including having a basic helping orientation; being authentic, nonjudgmental, genuine, accepting, respectful, responsive, present, empathic, and supportive; and being willing to self-disclose when appropriate)
- An interest in the mind, not just behavior
- Curiosity and the not-knowing (inquisitive) stance
- Monitoring misunderstandings (alliance ruptures)

Note. MBT–C = mentalization-based treatment for children.

THE THERAPEUTIC PRESENCE OF THE MBT–C THERAPIST

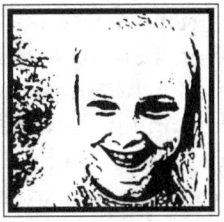 Seven-year-old Belinda started time-limited MBT–C because she was anxious, withdrawn, and had difficulty making friends at school. She has lived with her mother and grandmother since her parents divorced after years of arguing, shouting, and recriminations. Her parents felt that they had protected Belinda from witnessing this, but it was clear that Belinda's needs had been neglected amid the acrimony, and both her mother and grandmother conveniently saw her as a child who "just kept herself to herself and didn't need friends."

When the therapist first meets Belinda, he is struck by how little eye contact she makes. At their first individual meeting, Belinda follows the therapist to the playroom but sits rather listlessly, drawing circles on a piece of paper. When the therapist invites her to play a game of catch, Belinda looks surprised, but accepts. She throws the ball a few times, but her coordination is poor, and one of her throws knocks a plastic cup off the table onto the floor. Belinda glances quickly at the therapist and appears scared. The therapist smiles at Belinda and gets down to floor level, picking up the cup. "Don't worry—not broken," he says and shows Belinda the cup. Then he goes on: "I don't know what you're like, but when I go somewhere new, I'm always a bit nervous about what people are going to think of me. I don't know if they're going to like me or not."

Belinda looks at the therapist with a bit of curiosity. "Know the feeling?" he asks, but Belinda doesn't reply. Instead, she picks up the ball, and they carry on playing catch. The therapist starts adding in different tricks, and soon they are laughing. "Good catch!" he says, when Belinda reaches a ball that is quite high. And when he misses one and the soft ball bounces off Belinda's nose, the therapist says, "Ouch!" in a playful, somewhat exaggerated manner. "Did that hurt?" he asks, but Belinda shakes her head no.

In the opening part of this session, the therapist is not doing much that may look like mentalizing therapy. He isn't using any sophisticated techniques or trying to invite explicit mentalizing ("What did you think I was thinking when the cup got knocked off the table?"). Instead, he is acting like a regular person, meeting an anxious girl for the first time, in an unfamiliar place, just the two of them.

This natural, human therapeutic presence is at the heart of time-limited MBT–C therapy, just as it is for most therapies. Yet because there is always a danger that it gets overlooked or taken for granted, we begin this chapter by emphasizing the importance of this fundamental therapeutic presence. As Rogers (1957) described in his seminal work on humanistic (person-centered) therapy, this therapeutic presence includes *empathy*, *genuineness*, and *nonjudgmental, positive regard*. In his actions and behavior, Belinda's therapist presents himself as an interested, well-disposed adult, who engages with Belinda in a reciprocal way and shows interest in understanding how Belinda is feeling. He is not a "blank screen" but speaks about feelings and discloses a little of his own personal experience and what goes on in his own mind. The MBT–C therapist can answer questions from the child or parents as well as practice *judicious self-disclosure*. A survey of experienced therapists suggests that only a small minority make use of self-disclosure in their work with children and that few view it as contributing to the aims of their work (Capobianco & Farber, 2005). But as Taylor (2012) wrote, when working from a mentalizing stance, it is helpful to have "a clear, [but] perhaps a little flexible, boundary between the personal and the private domains" (p. 93) so that we can be genuine while at the same time mindful not to disclose personal information that we may not feel comfortable sharing. Speaking openly about oneself can often help engage children, especially in the early stages of therapy, and can help create a sense that the therapist is friendly, interested, and noncritical (Barish, 2009). In this way, the therapist brings herself in as a person with her own mind and perspective and models honesty and courage for the children and families she works with.

For example, when Belinda knocks the cup off the table, accidentally, her therapist first reassures her that no damage has been done and, implicitly, that he is not angry and Belinda isn't going to be punished. He shows empathy with how Belinda might be feeling but also behaves in a supportive way. He isn't detached, aloof, or inscrutable, but as Fonagy and Bateman (2006) advised, neither is he bubbling over with emotion in a way that might overwhelm the child. He is helping to create a (relatively) safe context in which levels of arousal can be modulated (neither too high nor too low) and in which there are two human beings in the room, both with their own thoughts, feelings, and histories. Both are probably anxious, and both expectant.

Fonagy and Allison (2014) described MBT for adults as a means of "establishing epistemic trust in relation to social learning in an attachment context" (p. 372). In other words, the relationship with a therapist, when there is a sufficient level of relational safety, offers an opportunity for the individual to "consider new knowledge from another person as trustworthy, generalizable, and relevant to the self" (Fonagy & Allison, 2014, p. 373). This, they suggested, is only marginally important in terms of the particular content that individuals may learn within the therapy itself (e.g., a new way of understanding why they have always been scared of meeting new people). Instead, the real significance lies in the fact that the *reduction in epistemic vigilance* brings about change in rigidly held beliefs and opens up the capacity for "social learning," that is, the possibility of having different kinds of interactions and experiences in the world. This in turn helps changes that have taken place within therapy to be sustained beyond therapy.

All of this is perhaps just a sophisticated way of saying that the therapeutic presence of the adult who is offering MBT–C is a crucial element, and we should not underestimate the importance of this personal quality. It is not a set of fixed behaviors, because each of us is different, so that being jokey for one therapist might convey authenticity, whereas for another, it would be forced and unnatural. These individual differences can easily be accommodated in MBT–C; what is important is the sense the child gets of being with an adult who is genuine, nonjudgmental, empathic, and comfortable with a certain level of self-disclosure. Given what we know from developmental research (e.g., Schore, 1994) about the role of positive affect, including joy and delight, in normal child development, it is perhaps not surprising that we share Barish's (2009) view that the therapist's "enthusiastic responsiveness" to a child's own interests is a key, but neglected, element of work with children. This in itself may not be sufficient for therapy to be effective, but without it, the chances of success are certainly much slimmer.

AN INTEREST IN THE MIND, NOT JUST BEHAVIOR

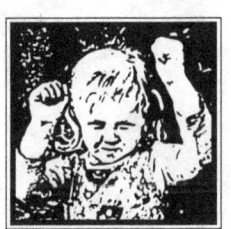 Anne, who is 6 years old, is sitting at a low table, intensely focused on a set of farm and wild animal toys in front of her. Her therapist is sitting at a right angle to her on a low chair, so that she is close by but not intruding on Anne's space. On the table, a flock of sheep huddle behind a fence, and Anne is holding a lion. "You be the sheep!" Anne demands excitedly, as she stealthily moves the lion across the table, letting out a low growling sound. As she does so, she looks up at her therapist, with a look of pleasure on her face. Her therapist's eyes widen, with an exaggerated look of shock at the growling sound, although her face and eyes glint, showing pleasure in the game.

The therapist picks up one of the sheep and lets out a "baa-ing" sound, then moves the sheep backward, fearfully. "Oh no! Here comes that nasty lion—I hope it's not going to eat me!" she says. Anne enjoys this and moves her lion forward in a menacing way, this time letting out a full roar. The therapist now does an exaggerated "Aaaagh! I'm scared!

Help me!" and notices that Anne glances up at her face, as if checking to see whether this is real fear or just pretend. Seeing it is playful, she roars again.

After repeated scenes in which Anne takes pleasure in the lion intimidating the sheep, the therapist tries to introduce some more flexibility and a potentially protective figure, bringing in a dog that she places in front of the sheep, as if protecting them (see Figure 4.1). "Grrrrr," she says, assuming the dog's voice, "I'll keep you safe."

At this, Anne immediately lashes out and flicks the dog off the table, turning to her therapist with a look of anger. "No!" she yells, "that's not in the game!"

Her therapist, somewhat taken aback by the force of Anne's reaction, leans back a little, then says, "I'm sorry, Anne, I got it wrong!"

Anne's mood slightly softens, but she still looks displeased. The therapist says, in an exaggerated voice, with her eyebrows furrowing together: "Oh, it is soooo annoying when grown-ups get it wrong! I feel so cross!"

Anne repeats, "You got it wrong!"

"Yes," replies the therapist, now looking away, in a way that demonstrates she's reflecting to herself on what happened. "I didn't mean to spoil the game, but I can see now that you may have felt a little frustrated when I put the dog there. I wonder why I did that . . . ?"

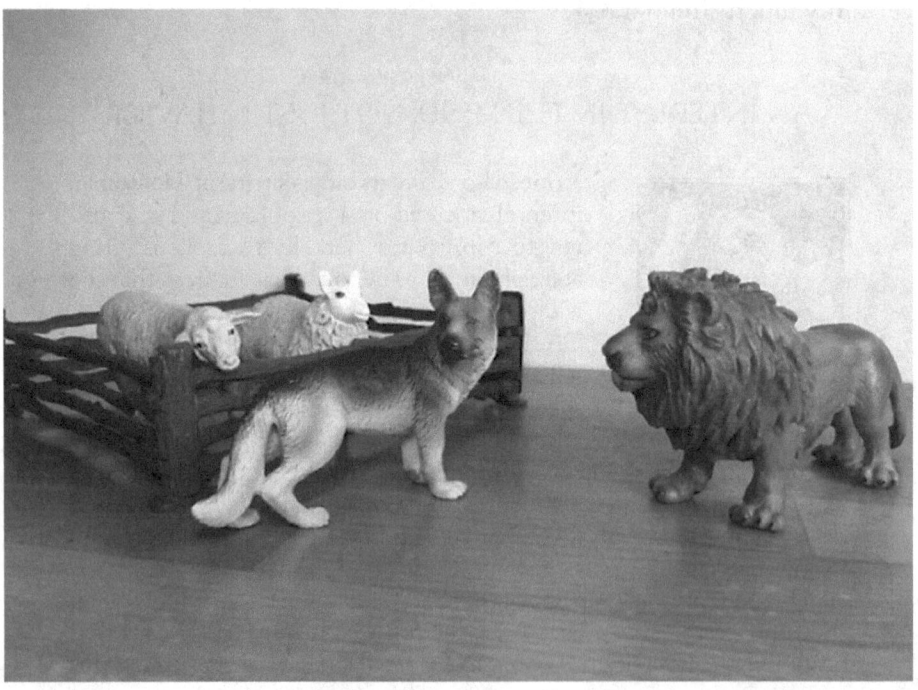

Figure 4.1. The toy animals used in Anne's play.

In the first chapter, on the developmental origins of the capacity to mentalize, we spoke about the way in which an infant's sense of affective self is built up through repeated experiences of *contingent responses and marked mirroring*, so that what starts out as a set of undifferentiated tension states can gradually be transformed into second-order representations of affect states—for example, an awareness of being "angry," rather than some undifferentiated, negative state of tension. We described how, over time, this helps to establish an ongoing sense of an *affective self*—one that can develop a certain level of self-control because emotions are not simply experienced, in an undifferentiated, potentially overwhelming way. Gergely and Watson (1996, 1999) have described the process through which this gradually happens as the social biofeedback theory of parental affect-mirroring and emphasized the importance to this process of ostensive cues, contingent responsiveness, and marked mirroring.

For many of the children who are referred for time-limited MBT–C, there may be limitations in the degree to which they have established second-order representations of affective self-states, resulting in their lacking a capacity to manage strong emotions. They may not have had a sufficient experience of being responded to as a child with a mind, and as they grow older their increasingly challenging behaviors (often developed as a way of managing uncontained emotional states) further invite controlling or punitive responses on behalf of the adult (e.g., "If you do that again, then I'm going to have to ground you for 2 weeks!").

In time-limited MBT–C, as in many other forms of child therapy, pretend play can be an opportunity for continuing (or beginning) a process of helping children to develop a sense of themselves as a person with a mind, by finding themselves in the mind of the therapist. Although not all children referred for MBT–C have a capacity for pretend play, Anne is able to make use of play as a means of expressing some internal experience, while maintaining an awareness that the play is "not for real." When Anne's therapist joins in the play with the sheep and the lion, she is using, in a form that is developmentally appropriate for Anne, many of the *ostensive cues* that parents use with infants in the process of social biofeedback. These include appropriate eye contact (enough to stay engaged but not too much to be overwhelming); raising the eyebrows in a quizzical or inquiring way; changes in vocal tone (especially to mark emotional states as pretend); and shifts in posture, such as tilting the head or looking up in the distance to mark the act of reflection. The therapist can use an exaggerated (and sometimes slowed-down) voice to help make clear that she is not actually experiencing these emotions (e.g., the sheep's fear) but is presenting them back to the child in what Gergely and Watson (1996) described as a "saliently marked manner." Anne's attentive look at her therapist's face when she first voices her fear ("I'm scared!") demonstrates the vulnerability that children like her may experience when they find expressions of emotion overwhelming, that is, when the as-if quality is lost and they are experienced as real. This is the value of the pretend play, in which the whole setting is marked as make-believe, allowing the exploration of a range of affective states that might otherwise be felt as too intense, too immediate.

When the pretend play breaks down, as it did for Anne when her therapist introduced the protective dog, the therapist's first response was not to focus on Anne's behavior or to try to help Anne learn more appropriate ways to engage in reciprocal play. If the therapist had done so, she is likely to have fallen into a *nonmentalizing vicious circle*, as described in Chapter 2, in which a child's nonmentalizing actions are met by equally nonmentalizing responses. However, Anne's therapist also avoided what might appear to be a more mentalizing response, such as trying to talk about why Anne behaved in that way. As Bateman and Fonagy (2006) pointed out, forcing people to try to think about why they behaved in a certain way when they have just acted out (whether throwing a toy or attempting self-harm) is almost never productive,

> Rather, it forces them to focus on the behavior they engaged in that itself is a consequence of a failure of mentalization. The mentalizing therapist knows that this is precisely what the patient is incapable of doing: finding and giving a reason for their action. (p. 107)

When Anne knocks the toy dog off the table (breaking the play in a nonmentalizing state), the therapist's primary aim is to try to help down-regulate the affect because without achieving this, there is little chance of moving toward more mentalizing interaction. But as Gergely and Watson (e.g., 1996) have emphasized, the marked mirroring of negative affect states is especially important in the development of the self, and so the therapist also uses an exaggerated voice to name the cross feeling (being careful to take on the first person—"I feel cross"—rather than directly saying to Anne that *she* was cross, which might again have been overwhelming). Once Anne's affective state is more modulated, the therapist can go one step further, introducing the idea of an intentional state of mind ("I didn't mean to spoil the game.") and invite curiosity about why the therapist's own behavior evoked such a powerful reaction from Anne. Rather than focusing on Anne and her mind, the therapist shows some curiosity about her own mental states ("I wonder why I did that?"), inviting Anne to be curious about why the therapist decided to introduce the dog into the game at that particular moment. The focus, then, remains on the mind (of both child and therapist), and not only on behavior.

CURIOSITY AND THE NOT-KNOWING
(INQUISITIVE) STANCE

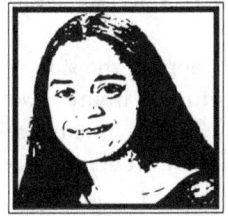 In the initial family meeting, the therapists are exploring different ideas about the anxiety that 11-year-old Liza has. Her parents don't think it is related to their frequent, late-night arguments with Liza's older brother, because "she's always asleep at the time." Her dad thinks that Liza may be feigning her anxiety to get attention; her mother says that she herself had been very anxious as a child, so it is "probably something genetic" and that she is sure Liza will grow out of it in the same way that she did.

During the meeting, one of the therapists explains that she doesn't know for sure why Liza gets so anxious, but she is really interested to hear the different ideas that people have. When Dad says that he thinks Liza is just trying to get attention, the therapist turns to Liza's mother and asks her if she has any thoughts about why her husband sees it that way. Liza's mom says that Dad doesn't like it when Liza clings onto her, especially in the evenings, before bed, when her husband wants to have a bit of quiet time with his wife.

"So let me check that I've understood," says the therapist. "Do you mean that he might want to be spending that time with you and gets frustrated when Liza won't leave the two of you alone?"

"Yes, that's right," says Liza's mom.

The therapist then turns to Liza's dad and asks what he thought about his wife's idea. "Yes, that's true I guess," he says, sounding a bit more thoughtful than he had earlier, "but I don't think it's just me who gets frustrated by it—my wife does too."

"How can you tell?" asks the therapist.

The father replies, "Oh, she's got a special face she puts on—you can always tell by that face when she's annoyed!"

Liza giggles, and the therapist turns to her and asks her if she knows the face that Dad is talking about. Liza nods, looking a little shy. The therapist asks Liza if she could show her what the face looks like, and Liza pulls a face—half quizzical, half cross. Both Liza's parents laugh, and the therapist turns to the mother and asks, "Has she got that right?" Liza's mother nods, looking at her daughter with some curiosity.

"Did you know that Liza knew about that face?" the therapist asks.

Mom says no but glances at Dad. The therapist notices this and says, "I just noticed that glance between you, but I don't know what it means."

The parents look at each other again, and then Dad says, "I think it means, 'I don't want to talk about this.'"

The therapist looks across at Mom, who then turns to the therapist and asks, "Is this really relevant? I thought we'd come here to talk about Liza's anxiety."

The therapist thanks her for asking this and says, tapping the side of her head, "Yes, perhaps I should explain what was going on in my head that made me ask. I can see that perhaps otherwise it may not make much sense. Let me see. I've only just met you. I guess we were all sharing our ideas about why Liza sometimes gets anxious, and it seems that there were different perspectives on what is going on when she becomes anxious and clingy in the evening. I guess I had a feeling it was important, wanted to follow this idea, and see where it led. But I did not have a preconceived idea. Would it be OK with you if we sometimes try following an idea to see where it leads us, even if sometimes it takes us to a dead end?"

While saying this, the therapist makes a mental note that Liza's mother may feel anxious about trying to meet her husband's expectations while simultaneously responding to Liza's needs for reassurance, and wonders whether this may make her less patient with Liza in the evening. She thinks that this is a potentially sensitive subject that may be important for the parents to discuss when they have their own meetings with the therapist.

When trying to define the essence of the mentalizing stance, a number of authors have rightly emphasized the centrality of not knowing. As Bateman and Fonagy (2006) were quick to clarify, describing the MBT therapist as taking a not-knowing stance is not synonymous with the therapist's having no knowledge or no ideas of her own. As mentalizing therapists, we are not expected to ignore our theoretical knowledge and clinical expertise, nor are we to refrain from forming our own hypotheses about what might be going on in the clinical setting. These hypotheses should, however, be seen as mental constructs, rather than absolute knowledge, and explored together with the child and/or parents in therapy. The not-knowing stance implies starting from an assumption that knowledge of the other (or indeed of the self) is not a straightforward process; we always have to work to try to understand the experience of others. *Being inquisitive*, as manifested in a process of active questioning, is a key component of MBT–C. This stance clearly has similarities to the approach taken by systemic practitioners (with the process of circular questioning), or indeed to the model of *collaborative inquiry* that is a hallmark of third-wave cognitive behavior therapy. What is specific about the mentalizing stance, however, is that the curiosity is specifically focused on mental states and how they may be linked to behaviors.

As Arietta Slade (2008) put it, when speaking about working with parents from a mentalizing perspective, in *being curious* the therapist is trying to model a reflective stance (p. 223), which can include

- struggling to imagine the child's experience;
- talking about feelings and linking them to behaviors;
- coming to realize that feelings change over time; and
- remaining aware that we can have a sense of what someone else feels but can never be sure we are correct, yet we can remain curious and open to discovering it.

One of the core features of good mentalization is this notion of the *mind's opacity*—that one cannot ever be sure of what another person thinks or feels. Allen, O'Malley, Freeman, and Bateman (2012) referred to it as "a non-judgmental attitude of curiosity, inquisitiveness and open-mindedness" (p. 160). The MBT–C therapist tries to avoid any sense of being an expert who knows better or knows for sure what is going on in the mind of the other. If you hear an MBT therapist start a sentence with the words "When you say that, what you *really* mean is . . ." you can be sure they are in a nonmentalizing frame of mind!

In most cases, taking on an expert position—giving advice or telling the patient what to do—does not promote mentalization. By modeling a not-knowing stance and stimulating curiosity and motivation to inquire into mental states, the therapist tries to help the child and parents become curious about the child's experiences and promote their understanding that they are separate from the parents. So when Liza's therapist starts exploring the different ideas that the family members have about Liza's anxiety, she is already marking these thoughts as just that: different perspectives, which are worth taking seriously, worth understanding better, but not absolute truth.

In this way, the therapist is working from an inquisitive stance based on the understanding that *mental states of others are opaque* and that when one attempts to imagine what the other thinks and feels followed by recruiting the other to figure it out, this often results in an improvement of affect regulation and the overall quality of interpersonal relationships. When Liza's dad first suggests that Liza is anxious and clinging just to get attention, the therapist doesn't directly challenge this idea; doing so might have led into a cognitive debate about whether Dad was right or wrong. Although the therapist may think this was unlikely to be the real reason for Liza's behavior (i.e., the therapist has her own ideas), by asking Mom for her views about why Dad saw Liza's behavior that way, she shows that she was accepting this view of Liza as Dad's perspective and implicitly modeling a view that there are probably good reasons why each of us holds the ideas that we do—reasons that can best be understood if we are curious about where they come from.

When Liza's therapist brings in her own perspective, there is a regular process of checking. The therapist tries not to assume anything with regard to feelings and reactions in the child or the parents but actively checks to see whether she has understood things correctly and uses the process of checking to acknowledge when she has gotten something wrong or to "thicken" (to use a systemic term) the narrative around a particular incident.

In this case, showing (and inviting) curiosity about the different perspectives that each of the family members has regarding Liza's anxious behavior seems to facilitate a more open discussion between the parents and create a more thoughtful and reflective atmosphere. However, at a certain point, the conversation moves to a topic that appears to make Liza's mother uncomfortable, and she challenges the therapist about why this is important to discuss. Once again, the therapist, rather than treating this as a manifestation of "resistance," uses it as an opportunity to try and spell out her own thinking, her own intentional states, that led her to take the discussion in this direction. The therapist makes clear that she does not necessarily fully understand the intentions behind her own behavior (our minds and intentions are somewhat opaque, even to ourselves). She uses this as an opportunity to share with Liza's parents her way of working but also, to build a more collaborative approach, to check how they experience this. The therapist, in a double sense, is trying to be *open-minded*, that is, "safe in [her] own failings and appropriately doubtful about [her] own viewpoints" (Fonagy & Bateman, 2006, p. 99), but also open-minded in the sense of opening up her own mind as an object of curiosity for the family. By tapping the side of her head, the therapist is actively demonstrating that what had been going on was a thinking process, one that she wanted to share with the family, but also one that she was curious to explore herself.

Maintaining a curious and inquisitive stance is both the simplest and the most challenging element of mentalizing therapy. After all, when working in a field in which we encounter children and families who may have experienced a great deal of trauma and emotions run high, the capacity for the system to become nonmentalizing should never be underestimated. So the MBT–C therapist will often investigate observed or reported interactions in a seemingly naive way. The therapist may mentalize aloud, entering the arena of safe uncertainty (Mason, 1993), sharing hunches and observations as she tries to understand what is going on. She might say, "I can see this makes perfect sense to you, but I'm not quite following. Can we go over that again bit by bit, so I can wrap my head around it?" *Slowing things down* is a powerful way to bring in new perspectives that might otherwise be missed.

One child, for example, was referred to a clinic because he was urinating everywhere, both at home and at school. The school was finding this behavior intolerable, and his foster parents had introduced a whole series of rewards and punishments, based on the assumption that he was "doing it on purpose" and needed to better control his behavior. Having not yet been fully caught up in this system of thinking, the MBT–C therapist took the opportunity, on first meeting with the social worker and foster parents, to show some curiosity about how this boy's experiences might relate to this symptom. After a bit of exploration, his social worker mentioned (rather matter-of-factly) that this boy had first been taken into care after a fire in his home, during which his younger brother had been burned to death. The therapist interrupted and checked to ensure that he had heard this correctly. The social worker stopped for a moment, and then said, more thoughtfully, that this was correct. "Gosh, what must it be like having that on your mind?" the therapist wondered aloud. There was a long silence in the room, but one that had a very different quality from the earlier, rather mechanical recounting of events. Somehow no one had ever made a connection between this incident and the boy's compulsive need to urinate. As they sat there, the faces of the social worker and the foster parent changed, and when they began speaking about the boy again, their voices had a different quality. They were now, to use a helpful definition of mentalizing, "looking at the other from the inside, and seeing themselves from the outside."

The following week, when the professional network met again, the foster parent reported that the urinating had stopped, yet no one had spoken directly to the boy about their conversation, and no new "strategies" had been implemented. As Sally Provence put it so well (as cited in Slade, 2008, p. 225), sometimes it is enough to say, "Don't just do something. Stand there and pay attention!"[1]

MONITORING MISUNDERSTANDINGS

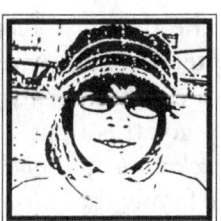 There was only one more session until the end of the time-limited MBT–C with Ruth (age 12). During this time, she had formed a close relationship with her therapist, and in this penultimate session, they were playing one of the games that Ruth had invented. As the therapist took his turn, Ruth took out her mobile phone and started filming what was happening. Her therapist felt suddenly anxious; he told Ruth that this was a private space, and it wasn't appropriate for her to be filming. Ruth apologized, said she understood, and they carried on playing.

---

[1]It should be added, to be clear, that MBT–C does not often lead to these kinds of "miracle cures" and that the process of change is as slow, messy, and gradual in MBT–C as in any other effective therapy!

When the session was over, the therapist found that he kept thinking about what had happened. He talked it over with a colleague, who asked him why he thought Ruth had decided to film at that particular moment. The therapist thought about it and wondered whether it was connected to the sessions coming to an end and whether Ruth had perhaps wanted to find a way to "hold on" to the connection with him. He realized that he had been feeling quite bad about holding the firm line on ending therapy because he knew that Ruth liked coming to see him. At the same time, he also recognized that she had made good progress and that stopping at this point was probably appropriate. He was going to miss her, however; he had enjoyed working with Ruth.

In using this supervisory space to reflect on his response to Ruth and be curious about what had motivated her to take out her camera at that point, the therapist felt that he had made a mistake in stopping her from filming. Although he was simply following his usual rules, in this case, he felt that his anxiety had made him overlook what might have been in Ruth's mind. So the following week, when he saw Ruth for their last meeting, the therapist went back to what had happened and apologized to Ruth, saying that he thought he had perhaps been a bit hasty in how he had responded and that he had wondered whether there might have been a good reason why Ruth had wanted to film them together. This led to an unusually open discussion between them about what it was like to have to say goodbye to people just as you were getting to know and like them. The therapist then wondered if they could go back and think how they could create a record of what they had shared together. Together they decided to make a photo record of some of the important things they had done together, and Ruth agreed that this was something that she would keep at home but not put online. The central image was a "selfie," of Ruth and her therapist standing together, holding a game that they had often played.

When working from the not-knowing stance, the therapist keeps an open mind to the fact that there are times (quite often, in fact) when we may not understand things correctly. Sometimes this can be quickly dealt with by the simple act of checking: "Let me see if I got this right." Even more important is to model honesty and openness, by *acknowledging one's own misunderstandings*. The therapist tries to convey to the family that misunderstandings are great opportunities to revisit an event or action to learn more about contexts, experiences, and feelings.

When Ruth's therapist asked her to stop filming in their session, this was not a mistake in any absolute sense; it is clearly appropriate to have certain rules about what can and cannot happen in a therapy room, and there are good reasons why as therapists we might not want to find a video of ourselves in session appearing on YouTube or Facebook. But from a mentalizing perspective, it is possible to see what happened in this interaction as a mistake or a misunderstanding on the therapist's part, insofar as he had probably mistaken the intention behind Ruth's actions and so had quickly moved to controlling her behavior (asking her to erase the video and put away her phone), rather than holding on to a curiosity about what had made her start filming in the first place.

That the therapist had slipped into a nonmentalizing response is perfectly understandable in this context, if we remember that all of us struggle to mentalize when our anxiety-levels are raised. For the therapist at this moment, seeing the camera not only raised professional anxieties about boundaries and confidentiality but probably also linked to his own difficult feelings about ending the therapy and his struggle to acknowledge the depth of loss that Ruth was likely to feel about this significant relationship. As do we all, the therapist benefitted from having a space and time to reflect on this, and his colleague did an inspired piece of mentalizing supervision when she avoided telling the therapist how he *should* have handled the situation, but instead invited him to be curious about Ruth's mental state at the moment that she took out her camera phone. In doing so, the therapist was able to better regulate his own emotions and could also become more curious about his own emotional reactions, some of which related to his specific relationship with Ruth and some to his more personal feelings about his professional competency: How would people look at him if they saw that he was "just playing" in sessions with a child?

Once his capacity to mentalize had been reestablished, Ruth's therapist was ready to acknowledge this misunderstanding and apologize to Ruth for his hasty response. Such apologies, when genuine, can be a powerful component of the mentalizing stance because they model a way of being in which we are able to reflect on what has happened and acknowledge that we can all get things wrong when we aren't able to mentalize. It introduces a model of *rupture and repair*, which Schore (e.g., 1994, 2003), among others, has shown to be central to the development of the early parent–infant relationship, just as Safran and Muran (2000) and others have shown its centrality to building a therapeutic alliance in work with adults.

In acknowledging his error and showing an interest in going back and understanding what had been going on in Ruth's mind the previous week, the therapist also contributed to creating a safe enough space for a different kind of discussion to take place, one in which the experience of loss, so central to Ruth's life, could be thought about and put into words, rather than simply repeated. The therapist was able to share with Ruth some ideas he had about why she may have wanted to film them, but he did so from a not-knowing position, simply sharing his ideas as one perspective. He was also able to reflect with Ruth on his own emotional reaction and how it led him to react in a controlling way ("I think I felt a bit put on the spot and didn't feel comfortable, so I just wanted to make it stop—by telling you to stop!").

Some might question whether it was really necessary to then actually allow Ruth to take photos in the room. Certainly, there is a teleological quality to this ("I can remember you because I've got a photo to prove it"), but as Bateman and Fonagy (2006) pointed out, in work with adults with borderline personality disorder, sometimes "being kept in mind has to be manifest in physical reality" (p. 96). For children whose capacity to symbolization is still fragile, there may be times when the mentalizing therapist is also the *doing therapist*, finding concrete ways to help the child feel that they are kept in mind—and are able to keep the other in mind, too. Ruth was a child who already had a certain capacity to recognize thoughts and feelings and reflect on how they might be linked to behaviors. When the therapist first asked her to stop filming, she was able to self-regulate and carry on as if unaffected. (In fact, we could say that she was overregulated, like many children who have a pattern of dismissive attachments.) However, when working with children who have rarely been seen as separate individuals by their caregivers, the misunderstandings, mistakes, and alliance ruptures can be far more dramatic. It is not uncommon for the therapist to feel provoked by a child's behavior and then reject the child. Although it is not always easy to do so in the moment, the way to handle these situations as a mentalizing therapist is to take responsibility for any misunderstandings and mistakes and to return to the not-knowing stance. By taking responsibility for the interaction, the therapist validates the child's experience. By admitting not knowing, the therapist normalizes and models an understanding of the opacity of minds.

Quite often, the mentalizing therapist might find themselves taking responsibility for a mistake long before they understand what they have actually done:

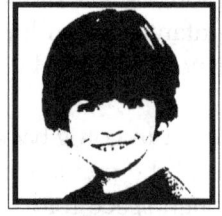 Mohammed (age 7) is only just starting his time-limited course of MBT–C when his therapist learns just before a session that Mohammed has been temporarily excluded from school because of an incident in which he had tried to poke another child in the eye with a pencil. Mohammed's father, who has been called away from work in the middle of the day to take him home, is extremely angry about what happened and arrives at the session in a very bad mood. He insists on joining the meeting, but the therapist suggests that she first have a bit of time alone with Mohammed. She would then invite Mohammed's father to join them a little later.

The therapist begins the session with Mohammed, who at first makes no reference to what had happened that day but begins a game in which a doll is being picked on by all the other dolls. At one point the doll kicks back and tells the others to go away. The therapist says, with some feeling: "It seems like she wants them all to get out of her face!" Mohammed turns round, abruptly, and throws the doll toward the therapist's face, at the same time screaming at her, "I hate you! I hate you!"

The therapist has not expected this and immediately moves backward, away from Mohammed, breaking eye contact. As she does so, she says, "Mohammed, I'm really sorry. I'm not quite sure what I've done, but I can see that I've really upset you. I'm so sorry." At that point, Mohammed bursts into tears.

When Mohammed's therapist apologized in this way, she had no idea what it was about her words that had produced such a violent reaction. The first step, from a mentalizing perspective, is simply to acknowledge that something the therapist has done had affected the child, and for that she was genuinely sorry. The tone of her voice made this absolutely clear, and by breaking eye contact, she was trying to help reduce the emotional intensity of the situation. To have tried to guess what it was in Mohammed's mind that had provoked this reaction might be seen as a mentalizing response (curiosity about mental states), but it would most likely have been entirely ineffective, given that the capacity for explicit mentalization is almost certainly lost when affect is this high. The first priority, when working in MBT–C, is to help regulate the emotional temperature, and at this point the therapist's apology was simply an acknowledgment that something had gone wrong between them and that the therapist hadn't intended to do this.

It was some time before Mohammed's therapist actually came back to this interaction, and she never fully came to understand what it was that had provoked his powerful emotions. But simply in going back to the event, the therapist demonstrated to Mohammed her wish to understand the intentional states underlying behavior and modeled a stance that misunderstandings offer opportunities to revisit to learn more about contexts, experiences, and feelings. One of our colleagues in the field of MBT with children and young people, Dickon Bevington (personal communication), goes as far as telling the adolescents he works with, in their first meeting, that he is almost certainly going to misunderstand them and make mistakes during their sessions. He asks them, if they can, to let him know when he's got something wrong, explaining that he won't always realize it himself. (The opacity of minds: We don't always realize when we've said or done something that has upset someone else.) And he adds, "I hope my next mistakes will not be hurtful but will give us a chance to take a step back and learn how to talk about how to work out our mistakes, misreadings, and any resulting hurt and anger."

USING SUPERVISION TO SUPPORT
THE MENTALIZING STANCE

In MBT–C, we try to help parents and children understand themselves and each other better by offering a therapy in which they learn a way to explore and talk about thoughts and feelings that helps them to be better attuned. For the therapists working with this model, it is equally important to actively mentalize and to notice when our mentalizing (inevitably) breaks down. In some clinics, therapists will be working in larger teams, and in some settings, the therapist may work with a single colleague or even alone. The most important factor, regardless, is to create a working environment that is safe and secure to allow mental states to be explored from a curious, not-knowing position. When we as therapists feel safe and supported, we are usually better able to ask for help and speak freely about experiences while working with challenging clients (Muller, 2009). However, a sense of safety is not always easy to maintain. We may work in an organization that sets prerequisites for our work that may not always be completely congruent with our ideals. Furthermore, different patients will challenge our capacity to remain reflective, and some children or families may trigger feelings and conflicts in the therapist that affect his or her mentalizing capacity.

One of the main tools therapists use to maintain their ability to reflect and stay on track is supervision. The therapist's supervision needs to provide a place of psychological safety, where the therapist can bring doubts, anxieties, thoughts, and anger and, last but not least, celebrate the work they do and the progress their patients make. Reflective questions about the therapist's own assumptions and beliefs can be helpful to unravel implicit aspects of the relationship between the therapist and the child and parents. When making the work explicit in a supervising context, aspects that are not directly observable can be discovered. It can also be important to reflect on cultural, family, or personal issues that might affect the relationship.

Given that most therapists work in relatively high-stress conditions and that much of what goes on in therapy happens in physical isolation behind closed doors, it is not surprising that the mentalizing stance can be hard to sustain for therapists. As Bevington and Fuggle (2012) noted, there can be "a tendency to move into non-mentalizing states such as teleological thinking (preoccupation with what to do) or with psychic equivalence (the belief that how the worker thinks/feels is actually how it is)" (p. 176). In light of such (normal) challenges, Bevington and Fuggle proposed a particular format for supervision that draws on our natural capacity to regain our capacity to mentalize through contact with trusted and supportive figures, while avoiding the risk that supervision becomes a simple narrative of dramatic events or an opportunity for the supervisor to demonstrate a "better" understanding of the child than the therapist. The latter, in particular, is likely to result in reduced mentalizing in the therapist, even when the insights about the child may be brilliant!

To keep the focus of supervision on maintaining (or reactivating) the therapist's mentalizing stance, Bevington and Fuggle (2012) proposed a four-step process, which they referred to as "Thinking Together":

- *Stage 1. Marking the task.* Rather than beginning with a detailed narrative of a session, the supervisor is encouraged to invite the therapist to briefly consider, "What do you need from this conversation?" This question, like time-limited therapy itself, can help to ensure that a focus is maintained in the supervision.
- *Stage 2. Stating the case.* The therapist is invited to share enough information about the case and the current situation without slipping into overly long storytelling. The supervisor helps the therapist to stay focused on the "simple bones" to avoid slipping into lengthy or overly detailed recounting of background history or what happened in the session.
- *Stage 3. Mentalizing the moment.* This is the heart of "Thinking Together," when the supervisor invites the therapist to explicitly reflect on the case and the issues that they have brought to supervision. The aim of supervision at this stage is not to find the "right" answers but to mentalize about the process, the child, the therapist, and their relation. It is important to find a balance between being self-critical and reassuring toward others or self. All clinicians have their own style, and it can be difficult not to become stuck in a particular stance or a single model but instead stay curious, open, flexible, and creative. Being challenged by colleagues in a safe space can facilitate an open-minded approach to our work.
- *Stage 4. Returning to purpose.* Having actively mentalized the moment and (we hope) helped the therapist regain their mentalizing stance, it is important to return to the task that was set at the beginning of the supervisory discussion, so that active mentalizing can be used to help address the issue at hand. Thus, this mirrors the therapeutic process itself, in which improved mentalizing is not an end in itself but a tool that can help us to develop more creative and flexible approaches to the challenges we face so that we are able to manage them better.

When thinking about our own understanding of the psychotherapeutic processes we engage in, we keep in mind that our own experiences and personal lives influence how we see, understand, and react to everything we encounter.

We have our own ways of seeing and interpreting things around us, depending on our cultures and histories. We also have our own bodily histories, with unique sensibilities that can become actualized in interactions with others. These subtleties are often difficult to put into words. Using video-recorded material can often reveal these interactions, as well as other implicit dynamics outside the therapist's explicit awareness. For this reason, we strongly recommend working with recorded material at least occasionally in supervision to be able to reflect on important processes that might otherwise go unnoticed.

Where possible, we have also found that it can be helpful to arrange the timing of sessions so that the therapist has the possibility of sitting down after the session and taking some time to reflect on thoughts and feelings in the moment. Going beyond writing summary notes for a file, we have found that it can be valuable to reflect on one's own emotions and bodily experiences. Often a lot of information is "hidden" in the interaction or felt by the therapist, which might be helpful to reveal the nature of the interaction with the child and the parent(s). For example, the therapist may note that they suddenly felt very sleepy during a session, for no apparent reason, or felt annoyed about something a parent said, when there was no clear logic for feeling like that. Noting and then reflecting on such emotional or bodily experiences (what might be called "the embodied counter-transference") can sometimes throw light on an important element of the interaction that at the time could not be fully mentalized.

CONCLUSION

In this chapter, we have tried to describe the therapeutic stance in MBT–C on the basis of four key elements: the therapeutic presence of the MBT–C therapist; an interest in the mind, not just behavior; curiosity and the not-knowing (inquisitive) stance; and monitoring misunderstandings. Several elements of this stance may be shared with other approaches; for example, there is significant overlap with the emphasis on playfulness, acceptance, curiosity, and empathy to be found in dyadic developmental psychotherapy (Hughes, 2004). What is specific about the mentalizing stance, we would argue, is the particular focus of the therapist's curiosity on *understanding intentional mental states*.

As a complement to this, Allen, Fonagy, and Bateman (2008, p. 166) helpfully presented a number of things that are not characteristics of the mentalizing therapist's stance:

- striving to be clever, brilliant, or insightful;
- offering complicated, lengthy explanations;

- making up an authoritative answer when you do not really know;
- assuming you know what the other is thinking;
- being rigid in your thinking; and
- focusing only on behaviors and actions rather than on the intentional states that underlie those behaviors.

All of these are forms of nonmentalizing, as described in Chapter 2. You may notice that most of these are things that therapists were doing at one time or another in several of the clinical vignettes described in this chapter. That is because all of us—patients or parents, therapists or children—lose our capacity to mentalize in certain moments, often because we are anxious, under pressure, or in some state of high arousal. All of this is normal and an inevitable part of clinical work. But the mentalizing therapist strives to notice when they are operating from such a nonmentalizing stance and (when possible) tries to become aware of these breakdowns in mentalizing and take steps to restore the mentalizing stance. Sometimes we may be able to do this ourselves, but often supervision, especially in the context of a secure relationship that can help to regulate our own levels of emotional arousal, plays an essential part.

It is because finding, losing, and reestablishing a mentalizing stance is so central to clinical work that we argue that the stance is the foundation of all therapeutic work in MBT–C. It may seem like a daunting task for a therapist to always be mentalizing, which is why it is important to underline that that is not the point and is not possible. No one can keep a mentalizing stance at all times. In later chapters, we discuss some ways in which the therapist can try to restore the capacity for mentalizing. But for now, we end this chapter with four points to be kept in mind when mentalizing seems hard:

1. You can enhance others' mentalization by doing it yourself.
2. When you are aware of nonmentalizing interventions, you are mentalizing.
3. Moments when mentalization stops (in you or in the child or parent) are possibilities for changes and new learning opportunities.
4. Just as we recognize that children develop a capacity for mentalizing in the context of relationships, so, too, can we as therapists use supervision as a form of relational learning to help us keep our mentalizing on track.

5

THE PROCESS OF ASSESSMENT IN TIME-LIMITED MBT–C

In this chapter, we describe a clinical approach to assessment, formulation, and the identification of a therapeutic focus statement and treatment goals in the context of time-limited mentalization-based treatment for children (MBT–C). This step is necessary to identify children who are most likely to benefit from this approach and also to develop a clear formulation that can help the family think about and understand the problem and how it links to the therapy being offered. Being clear and realistic about the focus and goals is an important start to working collaboratively with children and families and provides an opportunity to stimulate the mentalizing process. A specific emphasis is on the assessment of both the parents' and the child's capacity to mentalize and a formulation about how this is linked to the child's presenting difficulties. To provide a clear sense of how the different stages of

http://dx.doi.org/10.1037/0000028-006
Mentalization-Based Treatment for Children: A Time-Limited Approach, by N. Midgley, K. Ensink, K. Lindqvist, N. Malberg, and N. Muller

the assessment are linked, we present the assessment of one child, John, and his foster parents.

THE STRUCTURE OF THE ASSESSMENT PROCESS

There are different ways to initiate a time-limited MBT–C assessment, and it is important for the therapist to be flexible in how to respond to any request for help. Normally, the assessment phase will start with a family session, offered jointly by a child therapist and a parent therapist (when working in a pair), followed by two or three individual sessions with the child with parallel sessions for the parents. After these separate meetings, the therapists, child, and parents come together again for a review and feedback session where the outcome of the assessment can be discussed and a decision made about whether to continue with time-limited MBT–C (see Table 5.1 later in the chapter). The assessment may need to be combined with psychiatric or educational assessments or liaison with outside agencies that play a significant role in the child's life.

A joint meeting with parents and child together communicates a number of important MBT–C principles at the start of treatment:

- MBT–C does not work on the assumption that problems are simply "inside" the child,
- difficulties for one person are usually embedded within key relationships, and
- solving problems often involves work on the part of the whole family.

There are times when this format may need to be modified. For example, parents may feel that something is contributing to the child's difficulties (e.g., conflict between the parents, a parent's mental health difficulties) but are appropriately reluctant to discuss this in front of the child.

Whatever the specific format, the overall aim of the assessment in time-limited MBT–C is to develop a *mentalizing profile* of the child and the parents or family and to explore what links this might have with the difficulties that brought the child to treatment. If, at the end of the assessment, the child is to be offered time-limited MBT–C, the assessment process is also used to help reach an agreed focus for the work and set goals (see Exhibit 5.1). At the same time, the assessment process can be therapeutic in itself, offering opportunities for the clinicians to assess the child and family's capacity to make use of this particular way of working.

EXHIBIT 5.1
An Outline of the MBT–C Assessment

- **Initial meeting with child and family or carers**
  The therapists (when working in a pair) will meet with the child and parents together to learn more about what led to the referral and how each person sees the problems. At this session, the therapists make an initial assessment of the family's *mentalizing profile* and gain a sense of the interactions within the family.
- **Two or three meetings with the parents or carers**
  When working with two therapists, these meetings take place with the parents' therapist in parallel with the child's assessment meetings. They provide an opportunity to establish a therapeutic alliance with the parents and gain a better understanding of their perspective of the child and the presenting problem(s). During these sessions, the therapist formulates an initial assessment of parental *reflective functioning* (strengths and weaknesses) and how this may relate to the presenting problem(s).
- **Two or three meetings with the child**
  When working with two therapists, the child's therapist meets with the child to begin to establish a therapeutic alliance and gain a better understanding of the child's perspective. The therapist formulates an initial assessment of the child's capacity to mentalize (strengths and weaknesses) and how this may relate to the presenting problems.
- **Feedback and review session**
  In this joint meeting with both therapists, the parents, and child, the group reviews how the assessment has gone. The therapists share their formulations with the family. On this basis, a joint decision is made about whether to continue with time-limited MBT–C, and if so, to agree on the focus formulation and the treatment goals.

Note. MBT–C = mentalization-based treatment for children.

MEETING THE CHILD AND FAMILY FOR THE FIRST TIME

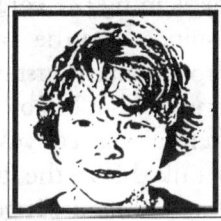

For the initial meeting, John (8 years old) comes with both his foster parents, Mr. and Mrs. F. John has been referred to the service because of severe aggressive outbursts and attachment trauma, and it is the first time he has come to the clinic. The two therapists who will be working with the family meet them in the waiting room together and take them through to the consulting room. They explain briefly what will happen in the first meeting. The therapist who is going to be meeting with the foster parents says that she has heard from the social worker that they are worried about the outbursts John has been having recently. But before she asks more about that, she wonders if they can begin by introducing themselves. Everyone nods, and the therapist adds that she has a slightly odd way of doing this: She would like everyone to select a toy animal from the basket in the center of the room that they think represents each person in the room. Would they be OK with that? Everyone agrees, with a mixture of curiosity and some apprehension on their faces.

When he is asked to choose an animal for each person, John begins by choosing a chimpanzee for himself. The therapist is curious about this choice and looks around the room to see if anyone has any thoughts about it. Mrs. F guesses he chose this because he can sometimes be quite cheeky, like a monkey. Both John and his foster father laugh at this, as if in recognition. When the therapist checks this out with John, he nods, but adds that chimpanzees also have sharp teeth. The therapist wonders aloud why that might be important to John, and John's foster father says that chimpanzees sometimes have to protect themselves when things don't feel safe. John looks intently and somewhat thoughtfully at his foster father, and then says that he wants to select an animal for his foster parents. Before he does so, the therapist suggests that each of the foster parents guesses which animal John might choose for them but not to say it aloud for now. When they've done so, John tells everyone that he has chosen a gorilla for his foster father. The therapist asks Mr. F if that was the animal he was expecting, and he laughs and says no, he thought he'd be an elephant! The therapist asks if he can guess why John might have chosen a gorilla, pointing out that gorillas and chimpanzees are both monkeys, but from different families. "They belong to the family of the apes, they belong to each other, but they also have their own family," John says with a lot of feeling. Mr. F responds to this in a warm and genuine way, gently putting his arm on John's shoulder and adding, "Just like us."

In starting with an initial family meeting, the therapists convey that they truly want to understand what has brought the family to seek help, would like to hear everyone's views and experiences, and will listen to these in a respectful and nonjudgmental way. One of the aims is to introduce the family to some of the components of a mentalizing approach, by both explaining the core elements of MBT–C and demonstrating the mentalizing stance from the start in the way the therapist interacts with family members. Throughout the first meeting, the therapists aim to develop a shared understanding of what has brought the child and family to seek help, representing the different perspectives that each family member might have. The therapists then link this to the family members' hopes and expectations about therapy. Seeing the family together also allows the therapists to observe something about the quality of attachment relationships in the family and to identify strengths and weaknesses in the family's capacity to mentalize together and to identify areas where the family's capacity to mentalize appears to be vulnerable. All of this is used to try to develop a preliminary formulation about the links between the family's mentalizing strengths and weaknesses and the issues that brought them to seek help.

A lot can be learned from listening to what family members say about each other, but much can also be learned by observing nonverbal, relational patterns between parents and child (Ensink, Leroux, Normandin, Biberdzic, & Fonagy, in press; Fonagy, 2015; Shai & Fonagy, 2014)—what Stern (1985) called their "ways of being together." For example, what parents do in interaction with their children and whether they are emotionally available, able to listen to and imagine their child's internal experience is as important, if not more important, than the parents' capacity to describe the child in an interview. These patterns of nonverbal, implicit relational knowledge (Lyons-Ruth et al., 1998) are important to observe in the initial family meeting.

The first family meeting is usually somewhat structured, drawing on ideas developed in the context of systemic and family-based MBT (Asen & Fonagy, 2012a; Keaveny et al., 2012), and can include the following elements:

- family introductions;
- clarifying how each family member sees the difficulties that brought them to seek therapy and what they have tried so far to address these problems;
- a family activity or game; and
- checking in and reviewing the session, then explaining what might happen next.

Family Introductions

First, each member of the family is invited to introduce one of the others and is asked to say a little bit about him or her as a person (e.g., what they like, the kind of person they are). Starting with this, rather than diving directly into the reasons why the child has been referred, helps to avoid focusing too quickly on the child and their problems. It also gives an opportunity—in a playful way—to discover something about the family relationships and introduces from the beginning the idea that the therapists are interested in different perspectives: to see ourselves from the outside, and others from the inside. While listening to these introductions, the therapist may want to keep certain questions in mind because this will help in the assessment of the family's capacity for mentalizing:

- Are the family members able to describe each other in terms of personal qualities, mental states and how they relate, or are their descriptions more concrete, focusing primarily on behavior?
- What is the emotional quality of the descriptions—are they negative, overly idealized, or nuanced?
- How do the family members being described respond to the description that others give of them?

After (or sometimes instead of) these verbal introductions, the therapists sometimes ask the family members to select an animal for each other and invite some discussion about these choices, looking for more implicit information about how different members of the family see each other and themselves (Muller & Midgley, 2015). As in the example with John and his foster parents, there can often be a playful quality to these introductions, with family members surprising themselves (and each other) with the way they are introduced or the images that others have of them. This can help move away from too great an emphasis on "the problem" and introduce the value of seeing other people's perspectives.

Finding Out About the Problem

After everyone in the room has been introduced (including the therapists, who can be asked to introduce each other), family members are asked about what brings them to seek help and are given the opportunity to express their own ideas about the problems that have brought them to therapy. There is a focus from the start on the idea that different people may have different perspectives and that the therapists are not interested in establishing who is right or wrong, but rather seeing how things look from everyone's position. Areas to explore may include the following (Asen & Fonagy, 2012a):

- *Focus on context and history of difficulties:* the nature and development of the problems; the contexts in which they present; how the family have tried to deal with the problem(s) and how they have tried to understand them; the effects on family and others; and history of previous treatment and help sought.
- *Explore differences:* find out whether family members might have different ideas about the difficulties or different understandings of what has caused them.

Often with younger children, the parents will talk about the child's problems, and the children may find it hard to speak about their problems themselves. However, they are also asked to give their views because they can often surprise their parents by showing that they have their own perspectives on the issues that brought them to therapy. The aim is to get a clear picture of the existing problems of the child, when and in what context the problem first developed, when it manifests now and what occurs, and the ideas everyone has about the meaning or history of the problems. Although the problems of the child are treated as an important topic, we also try to see the difficulties of the child from an interpersonal or systemic perspective and underline the interpersonal nature of the therapy, explaining that an effort will be made to find a way to address the problems together.

A Family Activity or Game

Where appropriate, the first session can include a family game or structured task, giving the therapists the opportunity to see how the family members interact with each other when carrying out a shared task. The therapists may introduce this by explaining that some families can easily *speak* about the strengths and difficulties they have, and some families are better at *showing* things to us by doing something together, so we always try to combine talking and doing things together. The activity suggested can be an interaction task, like "the squiggle" (Ensink, Leroux, et al., in press; Winnicott, 1996), in which the parent and child make a story together by completing each other's squiggles. A squiggle is a mark or beginning of a drawing started by one person, which the other person then completes and makes into a complete drawing. It provides an opportunity to observe whether the parents express an interest in the child's experience, can imagine the child's internal world, and are receptive to their affective communication and can elaborate and coconstruct a story with them that captures something that is of personal salience to the child. One could say that it is a test of the parent's capacity to imagine the child's experience, make it meaningful, and turn something that in the beginning is no more than a squiggle into a meaningful story with the child. Alternatively, the therapists can suggest a relatively free task, such as drawing or creating something out of clay or blocks, for example, asking the family to make their dream family house or a family zoo.

One reason for doing this is to see how the family members relate to each other in a play-based situation—the process of doing this is as important (if not more so) than what is actually created. In some families, especially where the initial interactions have been quite chaotic or where there is a lack of spontaneity, the therapist may feel that the family needs more structure for the game or task to be a good experience for everyone. The therapists may then choose a more structured task, such as asking the family to build a tower with a set of blocks.

Where the child and family give consent, and do not feel too anxious, it can be helpful to get permission to video-record the family task or game. This can be introduced by explaining that during a subsequent meeting with the parents the video will be watched together, to try to better understand the communication and relations within the family.

Checking In and Explaining What Might Happen Next

The first session usually ends with the therapists checking in with each person about how they have experienced the meeting. The therapists may also share with the family what they feel they have heard, check whether they have understood what the family has tried to convey, or if they missed anything important. The therapists will also discuss with the family whether they want to proceed and explain the assessment process. This is also an opportunity to explain something about what is meant by a *mentalization-based treatment* and what might happen next.

How one explains the concept of mentalizing will depend on the age and level of understanding of the child (and the parents), and there are different views on whether it is helpful or necessary to use the term *mentalization* with children or families. If therapists choose to do so, there is always the danger of becoming somewhat abstract or using too many words. Our experience is that it works best if you can link an explanation of the term to something that has happened in the room together, to a story from your own life, or to something that the child and family are likely to know. (If children have seen it, the Pixar film *Inside Out* can be a great way to talk about what mentalizing is.) Each person has his or her own style, but it can be helpful to start by saying something like the following:

> In our meetings together, you might sometimes hear me using a slightly odd word, *mentalizing*. This is a word we sometimes use as a way of trying to notice something that might be really helpful to you in sorting out the issues that brought you to therapy. *Mentalizing* is about trying to get interested in what might be going on people's minds when they say or do something. For example, I'm talking now, but you might be thinking "Why is he telling me this?" That's mentalizing, because you're trying to figure out what the intention is behind what I'm saying. If you get why I'm telling you this, things can make a lot more sense. But when we can't do that, or if we get it wrong, it can lead to all kinds of problems.

At this point (if eyes haven't glazed over already), it can be really helpful to link this explanation to something that has happened in the room or, failing that, to tell a story from your own experience. The story can be about how helpful good mentalizing can be, for example, saying to a child,

> Like today, do you remember when your dad said to you, "That must have been really hard when we left you on your own," and I noticed that a tear came into your eye and you gave him a big hug? That was Dad mentalizing well—he was thinking what it felt like to be you at that moment when you were left alone at the hospital, and I'm guessing that it made you feel good when he did that.

Or sometimes it can be about what happens when mentalizing goes wrong and why fixing it can be helpful. For example, you might say to a child,

> Do you remember how you told me today how angry you were with your dad because you thought he'd brought you here today as a punishment for behaving badly? And that made you sulk, then he started getting irritable with you? But when we all talked about it, your dad explained that the main reason he brought you here today was because he was really worried about you. Then when you understood that, I think it changed how you felt, didn't it? That's the power of mentalizing!

Once you've explained a bit about what mentalizing is and how it might link to the issues they came here to get help for, it is time to decide whether to continue with the assessment. Sometimes a family may want to go home and think before making a decision on whether to continue with the assessment. Often, at this stage, a sufficient level of trust has been built for the child to agree to meet with one of the therapists separately at the next meeting and for the parents to be comfortable with this. If they are not, then the structure of the assessment can be adapted; the important thing is not to follow an exact process but rather to keep in mind the aims of the MBT–C assessment and decide how best to achieve them in each case.

It is also helpful to contact teachers or other individuals at school to hear their thoughts and observations about the child. Sometimes children, especially those with trauma or attachments problems, behave differently at school and at home; as a result, they will most likely evoke different reactions that can help to inform the assessment (Muller, Gerits, & Siecker, 2012).

ASSESSMENT MEETINGS WITH THE CHILD

The assessment of the child is usually conducted over two or three sessions. The aim of these meetings is to develop a profile of the functioning and abilities of the child, their personality and way of relating, and an understanding of how the child's capacity for mentalizing may be linked to the presenting problems and difficulties. In addition the therapist will be attentive to areas where the child's mentalizing may be underdeveloped or situations in which an existing capacity to mentalize might break down. The aim of these assessment sessions is not just to give information to the therapist but also to create a relationship and a working alliance with the child. Rather than following a prescribed formula, the therapist uses their own creativity and clinical knowledge to find ways of engaging the child, selecting activities that facilitate a playful engagement and the opportunity to mentalize about self and other.

The therapist may decide to use both structured activities and free play. More structured tasks initiated by the therapist will give information regarding the child's ability to accept limits and follow instructions; free play will give information about the child's ability to handle lack of structure, take initiative, and use fantasy. Free play also provides an opportunity to observe whether the child is able to play and make play narratives with a beginning, a middle, and an end (Kernberg, Chazan, & Normandin, 1998; Tessier, Normandin, Ensink, & Fonagy, 2016), as well as identify traumatic play (Chazan, Kuchirko, Beebe, & Sossin, 2016) or whether there is play inhibition in which the capacity to play is disrupted.

Projective tasks can be incorporated for some assessments—for example, asking the child to tell a story using pictures, such as those used in the Thematic Apperception Test (Murray, 1943) or the Narrative Story Stems (Hodges, Steele, Hillman, Henderson, & Kaniuk, 2003). It may also be useful to use drawings, either by asking the child to draw different emotions or providing the child with drawings that are to be finished. In line with the MBT approach, during these sessions, the therapist uses his clinical judgment to actively respond and engage in play if this is considered helpful.

During the individual meetings, the therapist can express curiosity about the child's knowledge of why they have come to the service or whether they can articulate some of their problems using their own words. When children can express their own problems in a few words, it makes it much easier to find the right focus in MBT–C. Children might say something such as, "I am always anxious" or "I have no friends; no one wants to play with me," indicating that they consider that there is a problem and have a sense of what it is. At the end of the assessment phase, the therapist and child will try to agree on one goal that coming to therapy may be able to achieve and then formulate a *focus statement* for the therapy.

In addition to understanding the problem, the therapist should also try to look for the "vital spark" in the child (Winnicott, 1971b)—something that seems like a strength or a little burning flame that might help in the therapy. It can be something the child likes to do, is good at, or is curious about. This vital spark can be helpful as a source to go back to and maintain motivation when difficult moments in the therapy arise.

Assessing Attention Control or Basic Self-Regulation in the Child

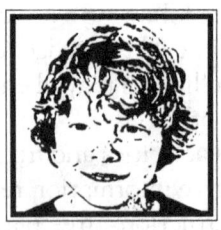
During his first individual assessment meeting, John has a limited attention span that is dependent on his own motivation. For example, when he chooses an activity himself, he can start playing and sustain it for a while but generally quickly loses concentration, being unable to complete activities. Activities suggested by his therapist are even harder to focus on, and he is easily distracted. He ignores the therapist when she asks him to do something in a way that seems similar to what the therapist has heard can be problematic at school and at home, with John not listening to instructions.

Sometimes during the session the therapist feels that John seems to not hear, either going into a dissociated state or simply tuning out. It soon becomes apparent that John has little ability to regulate impulses. He is also hypervigilant in the way he reacts very sensitively to sound. The therapist notices that John is listening to others talking in the adjoining room and that he is immediately distracted by the sound of doors slamming in the distance. Furthermore, time and again, he becomes disrupted by chaotic themes and emotions emerging from within—not contained and expressed in the play but actually disrupting the play. He can be playing peacefully, then suddenly there is a big crash, objects fly about the room, things get broken, and he genuinely seems not to have an idea of what is happening or a sense of being able to control it. In these situations, it is difficult to make contact with John, and attempts to ask him what was happening do not work. The therapist is aware that the same things happen at school, where John has sudden violent outbursts (as the staff perceives it). He cannot talk about it afterward.

Regarding his fine motor skills, the therapist notices that John uses the tweezers grip when holding the coloring crayons and actually has reasonably good fine-motor coordination while coloring and drawing. He is not yet able to write the letter J in "John" and inverts the direction of the little hook at the bottom of the letter J.

Making an assessment of a child's basic capacity for attention control and self-regulation is an important part of MBT–C. When there has been a good enough start in the early phase of life, children develop some sense of their body and skin, where their skin is a natural limit of the body, supporting a sense of an internal and external world (Stern, 1992). Being held and cuddled and offered physical comfort is a central part of parent–infant interactions but is also considered to underlie a feeling of being comfortable in one's body and skin. The first sense of self crystallizes around experiences of sensory stimulation, such as touching and being touched, hearing, seeing, smelling, and tasting (Stern, 1985), and forms the affective core of the self (Panksepp & Biven, 2012). This contributes to a sense of the embodied self and how one feels within oneself (Ensink, Berthelot, Biberdzic, & Normandin, 2016). Furthermore, mirroring helps the child pay attention to what is felt on the inside. However, some children who have experienced early neglect, like John, are not used to having a curiosity or awareness directed to what their body tells them. These children may have elevated pain thresholds (e.g., drinking hot chocolate without noticing that they are burning themselves) or reduced perception of bodily signals (e.g., difficulty recognizing when they are feeling hungry or when they need to visit the bathroom; Skårderud & Fonagy, 2012).

When children grow up in difficult circumstances (e.g., in an orphanage, with a parent who has psychiatric problems) and have had little help developing the capacity to put feelings into words, especially painful and difficult feelings, they frequently express feelings physically and act them out through their bodies. For example, prolonged institutionalization presents a set of risks associated with severe early deprivation and reduced stimulation that has marked negative effects on sensory, cognitive, and linguistic development (Johnson, 2000, 2002). Such children can be easily aroused and hypervigilant, which makes it harder to regulate their attention and emotions. They seem to be more focused on signals from the outside world. Therefore, the therapist tries to look for unusual reactivity to sound, light, touch, temperature, as well as disturbances in moving in space, gross motor skills, and fine motor skills. By school age, most children have managed to develop a way of attending only to important information and being able to cut out distractions from the environment by simply not paying attention to them. It is thus clinically significant when a child appears to be hypersensitive and distracted by everything around them. Being able to manage impulses from the inside is an essential basis that supports explicit mentalizing because there has to be room for mentalizing, rather than this getting drowned out by physical action (Zevalkink, Verheugt-Pleiter, & Fonagy, 2012). In other words, a child has to be able to endure a feeling without immediate action to be able to mentalize explicitly.

In exploring a child's basic capacity for attention control and basic self-regulation, the therapist keeps a number of questions in mind:

- Can the child focus attention?
- Can the child listen to others and to you?
- Does the child "live in their body"?
- Does the child have normal sensorimotor regulation capacity regarding sound, light, touch, temperature, movement in space, and gross/fine motor skills?
- Is the child hypervigilant?

Assessing Affect Regulation in the Child

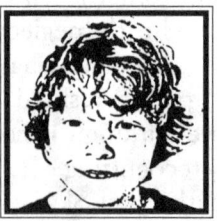

In the assessment session, John and the therapist are working with clay, and the clay lion John is making gets stuck to the table. As he tries to remove the lion from the table, it comes apart; John's face turns red, and he utters swear words. Despite his frustration, he shows that he has some internal control and also that he is able to accept limits. He shows that he takes pleasure in playing with water during the clay sculpting, but he holds back from doing this right away and waits for the therapist to give the go-ahead, seeking eye contact and asking for approval first in that way.

When John is emotionally touched by a topic, the therapist notices that he has difficulty saying why it touches him or what is happening inside. Instead, John shows it by wanting to do something else, standing up, or starting to talk about something else. When the therapist underlines his behavior by saying it might be painful for him not knowing where he belongs, he doesn't show a reaction. When he sees a seashell on the corner of a table, he briefly mentions that this must be a naughty shell, having to be put in the corner. When the therapist asks him if he sometimes has to stand in a corner because he has been naughty, John nods sadly.

During this brief interaction, John shows a range of emotions: frustration, sadness, and pleasure in what he is doing. He can express these feelings, stays in contact with the therapist, and does not appear to become overwhelmed by any one feeling. He is able to regulate some emotion by himself—for example, by standing up when he becomes frustrated and saying that he wants to do something else. However, he appears unable to identify and verbalize his feelings about his relationships with the key figures in his life. In these relationships, John expresses his feelings though behaviors rather than words and appears unable to put into words what he feels inside. Nevertheless, he is connected with what he experiences inside himself, while staying in contact with the therapist. The therapist notes that compared with her first session with John, she is beginning to feel that everything is there to start MBT–C as soon as John, his foster parents, and the therapists have agreed on a focus.

Other children have more difficulty expressing themselves. The therapist must then look for other ways of getting information about the child's emotional world. One way might be to read a picture book with the child in which all kinds of feelings are depicted and ask the child if they can recognize how the bear, fish, or child in the book feels. Perhaps the most important part, however, is to look at the child while they are playing and to ask oneself a number of questions to get some indication about their affect-regulation capacity:

- Which emotions does the child show in play or in the contact?
- Is the child able to play or use fantasy, and is this connected to the child's emotions?
- Which emotions does the child recognize or know?
- Which emotions seem to be difficult to express?
- How does the child handle difficult emotions in the session?
- What are the antecedents of the problematic behavior or antecedents of difficult feelings during the session?
- Does the child accept limits?
- Does the child ask for or accept help?
- Can the child be comforted when upset or accept positive remarks?

Explicit Mentalizing Capacity and Where Mentalizing Breaks Down

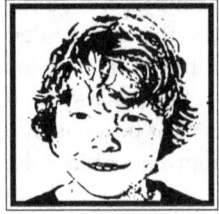

During this assessment session, John wants to play with the clay again. He starts making a bowl for his birth mother in the shape of a heart, saying it's because he loves her very much. He then wants to make a Donald Duck bowl for his younger brother (who lives with his biological mother), but while working on this, he starts thinking that the heart bowl could very well be for everyone. Looking at the leftover clay, John spontaneously comes up with the idea that he would like to make a bowl for himself. He wants to make the Donald Duck bowl for himself and not for his brother.

The therapist thinks to herself that for John, it is difficult that his brother lives with his biological mother, and he probably has jealous feelings about this. John tells her that the bowl he is making for himself must be very strong. He reinforces the edges of the bowl well. "It must be able to hold water—that's very important," he tells her.

The therapist wonders aloud whether John wants to become strong himself, not being angry all the time, being able to keep his feelings inside him. John nods and says that he worries his foster parents wouldn't want to keep him when he gets angry all the time. The therapist is not quite sure how "authentic" this comment is because John says this as if these may be words that someone has told him and he is just repeating them back. However, it could also be that he takes the feeling out of these words because he is really scared of engaging with the affects that the fear of losing his foster parents evokes in him.

To get a sense of the explicit mentalizing capacities of a child and their representations during the assessment phase, the therapist observes whether the child is able to think in mental state terms when describing self and others. The therapist should also be alert as to whether the child shows sign of any stable representations of self and others. When possible, the Child Attachment Interview (Shmueli-Goetz, Target, Fonagy, & Datta, 2008) can be used and rated with the Child and Adolescent Reflective Functioning Scale (Ensink, Normandin, et al., 2015; Ensink, Target, Oandasan, & Duval, 2015) because this provides an opportunity to obtain information about self and other representations, as well as mentalizing capacities. As a general rule of thumb, children in middle childhood should have some ability to think about themselves and others in mental-state terms rather than only in behavioral terms. If they are able to think in mental-state terms, difficulties in particular domains may be more easily addressed in short-term treatment since they already have some of the tools that may be useful here. When time and resources are limited, drawing on questions from the Child Attachment Interview, the therapist can ask children for three words to describe themselves and their relationship with attachment figures and then ask for an example of each adjective (e.g., "You said 'angry.' Can you tell me about a time when you were angry?"). The therapist tries to look at whether the child has a capacity for explicit mentalizing or whether they are able to think only in behavior terms. One aspect of this is whether the child is able to use some basic identification of mental states or has a more developed capacity to think in terms of mental states and link behaviors with underlying feelings and other mental states (Ensink, Target, et al., 2015; Vrouva, Target, & Ensink 2012).

The therapist is also sensitive to contexts in which mentalizing appears to break down because the therapist can then try to help the child become aware of this and develop mentalizing strategies specific to these contexts. In thinking about John, it is evident that he has the potential to mentalize, as seen in his play and the story of the gorillas and chimpanzees, but he does not yet spontaneously use mental-state language to communicate how he feels and talk about his predicament and difficulties as other 8-year-olds may be able to do. The therapist has the sense, however, that this can be achieved and developed with some scaffolding, and that in working with John, he could relatively easily develop a certain proficiency in naming his feelings as well as a mental-state language. The therapist also looks at the representations that children may have of themselves and their parents. For example, if John had an overly negative representation of himself, we would be concerned because in the contexts of normal development, children usually have largely positive self-representations (Target, Fonagy, & Shmueli-Goetz, 2003). Furthermore, if parents are represented in overly idealized or in split and polarized ways, with one parent idealized and the other described in extremely negative terms, this may be cause for concern and is noted by the therapist.

In the preceding vignette, John is able to use the clay to create some kind of representation of himself and others, and as such he shows some capacity for mentalization. However, it seems that this capacity may go offline when his attachment system is activated, for example, at the point when the therapist asks him about his worry that he may not be able to stay with his foster parents if he gets angry. Although John might appear to be mentalizing here, when he talks about his worry, the emotional quality of his words may indicate that he is operating in pretend mode—that is, the words are not really connected to a deeper level of emotional reality. It may also signal to the therapist that John feels afraid he will not be able to control his anger, so he might feel that he is bound to fail; this makes him anxious, and he wants to avoid talking about it. At the same time, he tries to use words but disconnects himself from his feelings when he does because they are too

TABLE 5.1
Modes of Prementalizing Thinking

Prementalizing mode	In the child we might see . . .	In ourselves we recognize . . .
Psychic equivalence (inside out thinking)	Play is often wild, chaotic, and destructive. The child acts as if he or she knows everything with certainty.	Feeling lost or confused. Noticing in oneself an inclination to set limits.
Pretend mode (the "elephant in the room")	The child's play has a rigid or monotonous character. The child is not in contact with feelings. Incongruent or low affect.	Feeling bored, start operating in autopilot. Feeling cut off or uninvolved. Finding your mind wandering or that you interrupt odd affects.
Teleological mode (quick-fix thinking)	The child demands a quick solution. The child demands that you do something NOW!	An intense wish to do something. Feeling controlled or under intense pressure. Starting to give practical advice or offer coping strategies.

overwhelming. One way that John's therapist becomes aware of this is by noticing that she finds herself rather unengaged when John speaks about his worry that the foster parents won't want to keep him, which is not how she usually responds when a child speaks about such an emotional topic. She wonders whether this might be because John himself doesn't sound entirely authentic—as if he is saying the words but isn't emotionally engaged himself. In time, the therapist may be able to help with this by explaining that it is scary to think that one may be rejected and lose the family that he is growing to love because of something he doesn't know how to control, such as anger.

Table 5.1 offers a description of a range of child behaviors that a therapist might see during an assessment, as well as some typical emotional responses that therapists may notice in themselves, and suggests how this relates to the various prementalizing modes that were described more fully in Chapter 2.

ASSESSMENT MEETINGS WITH THE PARENTS

A week after the initial meeting with John and his foster parents, one of the therapists meets with Mr. and Mrs. F on their own. They begin by reflecting on how the meeting had been the previous week and whether the foster parents have seen any reaction in John since then.

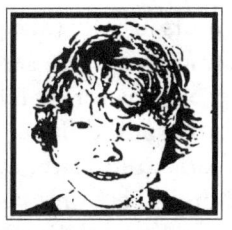 The therapist then explains that in this meeting, she wants to get to know them as John's foster parents and find out more about how things are from their perspective. She also reminds them about the joint activity they had filmed together with the entire family at the previous session and says that they will try to make time to review it in this meeting or the next one.

Quite quickly, Mr. and Mrs. F begin to speak about the importance of healthy food. After John visited his mother recently, he had told them stories about all the candy and snacks he had eaten. Back in the foster family, he had trouble eating normal food, which irritated the foster parents a lot because he spoke so extensively about everything he had eaten when he was with his mother. They tried to explain to him that the food his mother gave him was not really healthy and the food in their family was, and they instructed him not to eat too much candy while visiting his mother because of his weight problems. But after they had done this, they explain to the therapist, John stopped telling them about what he ate when he visited his mom, although they guessed he was probably still eating a lot of candy. Mrs. F speaks of her frustration about this and says she can't understand why John doesn't listen to their advice. "It is almost like he is deliberately doing it to upset us," she says. The therapist listens and empathizes with their frustration. She then says it sounds as if healthy eating is something that is really important to them. After further exploration, it becomes clear that Mrs. F had problems with being overweight herself when she was a child and is worried that John will be bullied in the way she had been. Her voice becomes softer as she remembers her own experiences.

At this point, the therapist invites them to think about whether John's reasons for eating the junk food might be similar to or different to the foster mother's when she was a child. Mr. and Mrs. F begin to think about how, for John, what he eats might feel like a question of which "parents" he is loyal to. Feeling sympathy with his situation, they think about whether they should stop talking to him about the unhealthy food and instead react positively to his enthusiastic way of telling and respond to his happiness about the contact with his mother. The therapist asks what they think this would be like for John. Mr. F thinks that he might be a bit suspicious at first and not sure if they really mean it. He remembers how John would often say, "Really? Are you sure?" as if doubting what they told him. But they think that if they persist, John might feel safer talking with them about how he feels. They decide to try to change their way of speaking to John, wanting to emphasize instead that there are differences in the way things go in the two families, but that it is OK to enjoy these differences. Mrs. F in particular recognizes that this won't be easy for her but that this is more her problem than John's.

The two or three sessions with the parents or carers usually take place while the child is being seen by a separate therapist, and in these sessions the therapist tries to make an appraisal about the problems for which the family sought help as well as the mentalizing capacities and difficulties of the parents or carers (Muller & Bakker, 2009; Muller & ten Kate, 2008). By that, we mean their capacity to think of children as separate people, with minds of their own, and to see the child's behavior (and their own, as parents) in terms of intentional mental states (Slade, 2007). During initial sessions, the therapist seeks to observe and listen for the ways in which the parents think about, manage, and try to understand and explain the child's behaviors and emotional states. The therapist should also be interested in the parents' own emotional reactions and their ability to reflect on those. On the basis of an initial assessment, the therapist can then define where to best try to meet the parents in terms of their current reflective functioning capacities.

There are several structured and reliable instruments for assessing mentalizing capacity in parents and carers, such as the Adult Attachment Interview (George, Kaplan, & Main, 1996) and the Parent Development Interview (Slade, Aber, Bresgi, Berger, & Kaplan, 2004). However, when there is neither the time nor the resources to use these structured interviews, certain questions that are part of these interview schedules can be useful in more clinical ways. For example, in the assessment meeting with the parents, the therapist can say, "Can you choose three adjectives that you feel reflect the relationship between you and your child? Does an incident or memory come to mind with respect to each of these adjectives?" or "Tell me about a time in the last week or two when you felt really angry as a parent. What kinds of situations make you feel this way? How do you handle your angry feelings?" Where appropriate, the therapist might also ask, "How do you think your own experiences of being parented affects your experience of being a parent now?" This last question helps the therapist to identify possible "ghosts in the nursery" (Fraiberg, Adelson, & Shapiro, 1975) or "angels in the nursery" (Lieberman, Padrón, Van Hom, & Harris, 2005), that is, traumatic or positive experiences from the parents' own histories that may be influencing the way they relate to their child. For parents who have experienced childhood abuse and neglect, being able to mentalize about these experiences and the impact they have had on their development and parenting appears to be particularly important in terms of child outcomes and relationship functioning (Ensink, Berthelot, Bernazzani, Normandin, & Fonagy, 2014). Sometimes, as in the case of John's foster mother, these issues may come up more spontaneously; but if not, there may be times when it is helpful to ask explicitly about them, while being clear why this is relevant to the issues that brought their child to therapy.

As in all aspects of MBT–C, the therapist tries to use the core features of the *mentalizing stance*, including empathy, curiosity, and an interest in different perspectives. When John's foster mother spoke about her frustration that John didn't listen to their advice on healthy eating, the therapist did not challenge her on this, and she avoided focusing on the behavior per se or whether it was right or wrong. When the therapist showed empathy with the foster mother's frustration, it seemed that she felt safer to speak about her own experiences as a child. Her softer voice was an indication to the therapist that the foster mother's mentalizing capacity was more "online" because the level of arousal had decreased. At that point, the therapist began to use some questions that invited explicit mentalizing: What did they think it would be like for John when they asked him about what he'd eaten with his mum? In what way might John's reasons for eating junk food be similar to or different from those of the foster mother when she was a child? By asking these questions, the therapist was encouraging the foster parents to take an inquisitive stance about John's mind and his experiences. For example, John's foster parents were able to imagine that when talking about food, John might feel as if he had to say which parents he liked best. But the word *might* was important—they did not express absolute certainty about this, although seeing it from this perspective helped them make better sense of the way John sometimes behaved with them. Features like this capacity to hold a position of *safe uncertainty* and be aware of the opacity of minds are helpful indicators of the parents' capacity to be reflective and sustain a stance of mind-mindedness (Meins et al., 2003), even in the face of their child's difficult behavior. Asen and Fonagy (2012b) suggested that therapists ask themselves the following questions as part of a "mentalizing checklist for parents":

- Does a parent feel the urge to speak for the other parent or the child in the family session?
- Do parents refer to their own thoughts or feelings?
- Do parents refer to feelings or thoughts of others in the family?
- Do parents consider the perspective of others?
- Do parents sometimes say, "I might be wrong, but I think she . . ." (opaqueness)?
- Do parents often use all-or-nothing or black-and-white words like *always* or *never*?
- Are the parents playful? Do they use humor?
- Are there special feelings or thoughts that seem to be avoided in the conversation or that often lead to escalation?
- When parents talk about their behavior, do they sometimes connect this to intentions?

Depending on their own histories, parents may vary greatly in their capacity to mentalize their child's experience, or they may be able to do this in some areas but be vulnerable to mentalizing breakdowns in others. For example, a parent may show the capacity to explicitly mentalize in the here and now, queued by questions from the therapist, or by reflecting on their own story as they tell it. The capacity to modulate, tolerate, and name affects as well as to empathize with the experience of the child is rooted in the capacity to reflect on one's own experiences, so if emotions are familiar and known to the parent, then they can probably recognize and respond to them in a coherent, organized, and meaningful way.

Parents with their own histories of insecure attachment may have more difficulty symbolizing the experiences and making sense of their child's communication, because the child's emotions can easily dysregulate them as well. To most effectively help parents who have their own histories of childhood trauma, special attention should be paid to understanding when mentalization breaks down and which situations are particularly challenging, even when they have good reflective functioning in general. For parents who have underdeveloped reflective function and cannot see beyond their child's behavior, the therapist may observe developmentally inappropriate, unpredictable, or chaotic and contradictory regulation strategies.

In this assessment meeting with John's foster parents, it was apparent that they were able to use the space provided by the therapist to explore John's experiences and to separate their own needs and wishes from his. In doing so, they were able to think about how they could best provide him with a sense of security and safety. As such, their capacity to mentalize was fundamentally good, but like for all of us, there were certain areas and contexts in which they were vulnerable to mentalizing breakdowns. At those points, Mrs. F seemed to operate in more of a psychic equivalence mode—that is, being sure that what was in her mind (about John) was how things actually were, out there. When the therapist recognized this and offered empathy rather than challenge, her capacity to become curious about John's experience and to imagine things from his perspective quickly revived.

This is not always the case with the families seeking help. As Fonagy and Campbell (2015) put it, therapeutic change for an individual child "can only be sustained . . . if the patient is able to use, and even to change their social environment in a way that allows them to continue to relax epistemic hyper-vigilance and foster their mentalizing strengths" (p. 245). However, when there is no safe haven at home, an intervention to take the child out of the threatening situation or to support the family's functioning might be necessary before thinking about treatment for the child.

GATHERING IMPRESSIONS INTO
A CASE FORMULATION

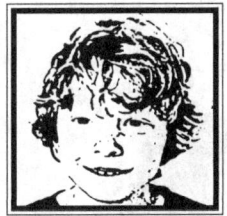 In their final assessment session, the therapists thank John and his foster parents for coming and ask them about their thoughts and feelings about the process so far. All three agree that it has not been what they expected, and when the therapists ask what they had expected, they say that they thought the therapist would be more like a doctor telling them what's wrong! The child therapist tells them that she's been thinking a lot about all they have shown and told her and that she has made a small story, which she would like to share with them. John looks pleased about this, and he leans in against his foster mother's body, as if waiting to hear a story at bedtime.

The therapist then begins: "There was once a little chimpanzee. He lived for a while with his mother in a group but had to leave her when he was really little, because she couldn't take care of him anymore. This was sad, because the chimpanzee hadn't learned all the words and rituals that are used in a chimpanzee family. After traveling around and staying in different places, the little chimpanzee came to a family of gorillas. This looked a bit like home, but sometimes he felt out of place and worried whether the gorilla family would let him stay. He often lacked the words to describe what he thought or felt. Sometimes he felt very alone because he missed his mother and because he had lived so long with others where he had felt like an outsider. Sometimes when he felt sad, he became angry, because it helped him feel a bit bigger. At the gorilla family, it often did feel like home, but sometimes it didn't. He was a chimpanzee after all. So he decided he wanted to find his own words and rituals to become stronger and not so angry anymore, and he decided he wanted to live with the gorillas and visit the chimpanzee family once in a while. The gorillas loved the little chimpanzee, and they were willing to learn more about how it is to be a chimpanzee." (Figure 5.1).

As the story ends, John's foster parents turn to look at him, and he smiles back at them. Pointing out the interaction, the therapist wondered if Mrs. F wants to let John know what's in her mind right now. She replies, "Just that we care about him a great deal and know that he's a lovely boy—even if he does sometimes drive us crazy!" This leads the therapist and the family back to thinking about their plans, and all agree that John should begin a block of 12 MBT–C sessions and that the foster parents will also attend, although they prefer to attend fortnightly, rather than every week.

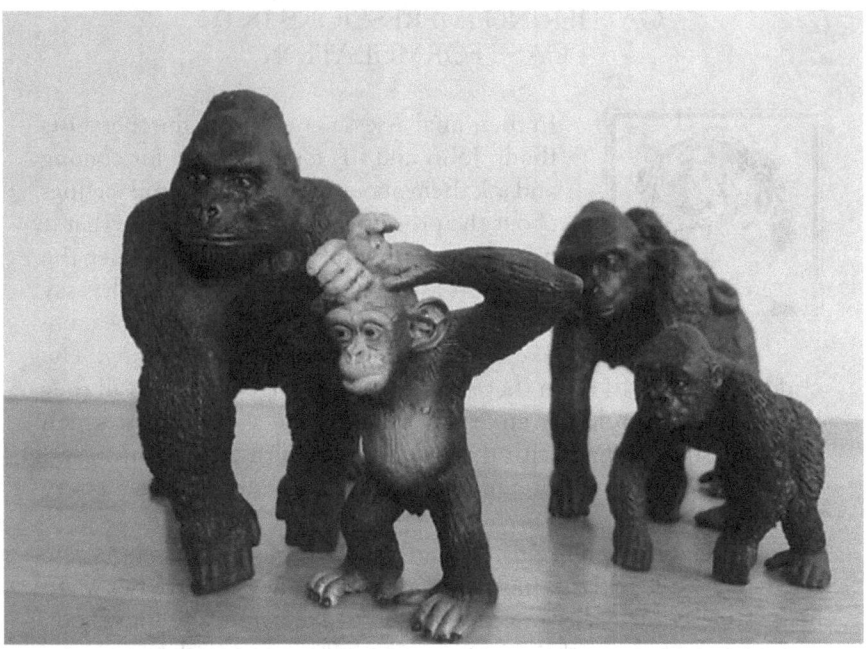

Figure 5.1. The animal figures John used to represent his family.

The final session in the assessment phase is usually with the parents and child together and is an opportunity for the therapists to share their thinking in a way that can be understood by both parents and the child. This shared formulation should ideally include the following:

- some thoughts about the mentalizing strengths in the child and family,
- some of the areas in which mentalizing is underdeveloped or may break down,
- provisional thoughts on how the first two points link to the issues that brought the family to seek help, and
- a recommendation about whether time-limited MBT–C could be an appropriate intervention to address these issues.

When putting together a mentalizing profile, it can be helpful to ask oneself, "How well can this person mentalize when at his or her best, and when is that?" and "How much difficulty does this person have with mentalizing when it breaks down, and when do such breakdowns tend to happen?" With this in mind, mentalizing problems can be put on a spectrum, with underdeveloped mentalizing at one end and specific or temporary breakdowns in mentalizing at the other.

Developing and coconstructing a shared formulation, as elaborated by Rossouw (2012) in the context of MBT with adolescents who self-harm, appears to be particularly useful. Rossouw pointed out that the aim of a formulation is "to explain the current difficulties in mentalizing and relational terms . . . [and] also to present to the young people and their families an image of themselves that will make them feel understood" (p. 137). The value of a formulation is also in its capacity to shape plans and give a focus to the work and to link the capacity to mentalize with the problems for which the family is seeking help. Sharing such ideas with children and their parents is not always easy, and it is important to avoid using overly technical language. A case formulation can be given in the form of a story, as the case example with John demonstrated, which can contain a metaphor that speaks to the possible implicit and explicit features of the problems, but it can also simply be a sentence or two.

In John's case, the therapist's assessment indicated that his foster parents had a good capacity to see John as a boy with thoughts and feelings, which could help them make sense of his behavior. Although there were areas in which their mentalizing capacity could break down, possibly because of issues derived from their own histories (e.g., the foster mother's response to John's not being careful about his diet and putting on weight), they were able to make use of the therapeutic space provided in the assessment to reflect on their own mental states and thereby separate out what belonged to John and what belonged to them. In doing so, they were able to think about John's loyalty conflict in a different way and modify how they responded to his behaviors accordingly.

Likewise, in his individual assessment meetings, when the circumstances were right, John demonstrated a capacity to regulate both his attention and affects. For example, over the course of the three meetings, he showed some capacity to regulate his emotions and make use of the therapeutic relationship to support this effort. He also showed some evidence of potentially being able to use mentalizing to make sense of his own behavior and the reactions of others, and he was able to engage in simple symbolic play, although the play narratives were not well elaborated, and to make use of the metaphor of the chimpanzee and the gorillas. However, it was also apparent that John's ability to mentalize was underdeveloped in a number of areas: He used little explicit mentalizing in his descriptions of himself and significant relationships. In addition, even the abilities he did have broke down easily when John felt anxious or afraid. It seemed likely that John's vulnerability to such disruptions was in part related to his early history, when he may not have experienced the type of sensitive responding to distress, mind-mindedness, and marked affect mirroring associated with the development of affect self-regulation (Fonagy, Steele, Steele, Moran, & Higgitt, 1991; Slade, 2005).

Given his many foster placements, John may have had few experiences of reflective parenting and caregivers looking beyond his behavior to imagine what it communicated about his internal experience. He may have had little support to articulate his feelings and concerns and develop self-regulation strategies. In short, John would have had few opportunities to experience the kind of benign interest in his mind that may facilitate the development of mentalizing with regard to self and others (Ensink, Bégin, Normandin, & Fonagy, 2016). Linking this to the referral, John's reported aggression and social isolation can be understood as a consequence of this vulnerability, and it was determined that a time-limited MBT–C intervention, with parallel work with his foster parents, could help him begin to strengthen these capacities, in the context of a therapeutic relationship in which he was able to gradually regain a sense of epistemic trust.

USING A FOCUS FORMULATION

The focus should be easy for child and parents to understand. Themes of the focus are often related to self-esteem, regulation, autonomy, dependency, and developmental forces. The focus formulation aims to be exploratory or affect regulatory and formulated in a nondramatic, even playful way. The focus formulation is different from a problem formulation in that it points to the work that can be done in therapy with an emphasis on hope, curiosity, and resources (Haugvik & Johns, 2008; Røed Hansen, 2012). The therapist can choose to formulate the focus as a short sentence or as a short story. When formulating a shorter focus, the therapist needs to explain more of her thinking, whereas a story can include more of the dynamics observed in the assessment, thereby being more self-explanatory.

Sharing the focus formulation with the family is one of the most important parts of the assessment; it concludes the assessment phase and introduces the treatment. When presenting the suggested focus formulation, it is helpful to explain the thinking behind your suggestion, thereby modeling how you can keep someone in mind, wonder about them, and think about them from different perspectives. For example,

> We've thought about you a lot and what a suitable focus could be. I thought about how you told us . . . and I wondered a lot about. . . .

When formulating a focus, there are some *focus traps* to avoid. The aim of the focus is to stimulate curiosity and mentalizing. However, some formulations can have the opposite effect. Contrary to many other models, a focus in MBT–C does not have to be well operationalized or easy to measure—in fact, it is actually preferable that it is not. The reason behind this is that we want to avoid a focus that makes it is easy to fail (e.g., "fight less at home," "dare to be more brave") because these are based on achievement or on unwanted behavior or symptom reduction (e.g., "worry less"). By contrast, the focus aims more at stimulating reflection and curiosity. Because we aim to look more at internal processes and not only behavior, the focus needs to be formulated with that in mind.

When thinking about John, his therapist suggested that a proposed focus formulation for the work could be: "What does a little chimpanzee need to be happy in a family of gorillas?" Sometimes the proposed focus does not feel right to the child or the family. It is important to offer the focus as just one option that can be negotiated, conveying the message that you are not necessary right, are not an expert, and that they can correct you or help identify another focus. Sometimes you might have to go back to the drawing board. It can be a constructive and therapeutic task to think together about what the focus should be.

For example, when discussing this case formulation with the foster parents, John's therapist noticed that the focus she had proposed concentrated more on desired changes in his behavior (and feelings), which perhaps reflected a pressure to try to sort out John's difficult behavior. Perhaps something more exploratory such as, "getting to know the chimpanzees and the gorillas better" or "finding out what chimpanzees need to be proud and happy" would have encouraged more of a sense of curiosity and interest in mental states and their link to how we feel and behave.

SETTING GOALS

It is increasingly common, when offering therapy to children, not only to use standardized pre- and postmeasures but also to make use of individualized treatment goals, such as the Goal Based Outcome Measures described by Law and Wolpert (2014). Setting a specific goal can help children and their parents focus on one central issue in a sea of problems. Progress toward a specific goal is both attainable and visible and can contribute to a sense of much-needed motivation and achievement, stimulating further change. It may appear as if such goal setting may contradict what has been said earlier about the importance of having a focus for treatment that is not behaviorally orientated. However, it is our experience that using goals and formulating a treatment focus can sit comfortably alongside each other, and both contribute to working effectively with time-limited MBT–C. The strategy also allows the child and family to set goals that are not easily captured by standardized outcome measures. These goals can relate to underlying factors, such as building confidence, resilience, and coping skills, which regularly appear as important targets for treatment when children and families are invited to set their own treatment goals (Jacob, Edbrooke-Childs, Law, & Wolpert, 2015).

Goal setting after the initial assessment should be clear and realistic and facilitate the ongoing evaluation process. When the therapists and family agree to work toward these shared goals, the chances of achieving them are higher, and the family is likely to be more motivated to attend treatment. Furthermore, specific and individual goals are helpful in evaluating the treatment and the process, as well as in making decisions about additional treatment. The goals set do not necessarily become the focus of the work in sessions but can be used as important indicators that the therapy is having a meaningful impact on the child and parents.

MBT–C is not primarily symptom focused, although it can be problem focused, but rather emphasizes the promotion of mentalizing and emotion regulation, and this informs the goal-setting process. When formulating goals, we recommend doing it on a relational and regulatory, rather than purely behavioral and symptomatic, level. On the one hand, if the goals set are too concrete, this may be incongruent with promoting mentalization. On the other hand, if the goals are too nonspecific, it will be difficult to assess progress and follow up as necessary, and it may not be clear to the family how the work in therapy applies to the difficulties that led them to seek help in the first place.

In the assessment phase, it is important to provide sufficient time to have a conversation in which both child and parents are present, and they can talk about why they have sought therapy and what they are hoping to achieve by coming to treatment. It should be clear to the child that the therapist knows about his specific problems and wants to try and help with him. When sharing the assessment, the therapist tries to share with the family, at a level that both parents and child can understand, a little about how they understand the problems in terms of mentalizing, regulatory difficulties, and family dynamics.

Where possible, we would encourage the use of goals jointly set by the child, parents, and therapist. When parents and children set goals separately, research suggests that parents tend to focus more on managing specific difficulties, whereas children also include goals related to personal growth and independence (Jacob et al., 2015). The process of jointly agreeing on goals invites discussion about the different views each person holds and so can facilitate a mentalizing process in itself, as the therapist and family members take on board each other's perspectives in trying to reach a shared set of goals. A shared agreement on goals can happen alongside agreeing on a focus statement for the therapy. These goals can, and should, be returned to at review meetings, at the ending of therapy, and during any booster sessions. It is our experience that the process of agreeing on goals can be as important as the goals themselves and that having this discussion upfront helps to reduce the likelihood of treatment dropout at a later stage.

CONCLUSION

In this chapter, we have described the assessment process in time-limited MBT–C. It is always important to complete a comprehensive assessment of the child and the parents in order to

- formulate a clear understanding of the nature and severity of the problems, their development, and key causal factors and maintaining factors;
- consider whether the impact on the child's functioning is specific to one area or is general and affecting multiple domains;
- develop an understanding of the child's and the parents' mentalizing strengths and difficulties and whether failures in mentalization are central to these;
- consider what treatment goals are realistic and identify the potentially most productive or central issue to focus on; and
- form an impression about whether the child or parents recognize that there is a problem, are motivated to find new ways of thinking about and doing things, and whether they appear to trust the therapist and thus be able to develop a good working alliance.

On this basis, the assessing therapist can decide whether it is appropriate to offer a time-limited, mentalization-based frame for the work and, if so, formulate ideas about the potential focus for the work.

6

DIRECT WORK WITH CHILDREN IN TIME-LIMITED MBT–C

In this chapter, we describe the main features of the direct work with children in mentalization-based treatment for children (MBT–C), including some of the techniques that can be used in sessions with a child. As we hope we have made clear throughout this book, techniques in themselves are only a means to an end, not an end in themselves. Their effectiveness depends on the quality of the therapeutic relationship that has been formed; the capacity to use the techniques in a lively and appropriate way, sensitivity to the "emotional temperature" in the room, and the child's level of functioning. In Chapter 4, we described the therapist's *mentalizing stance* and the role it plays as in all MBT work. This is the foundation on which the rest of the work can be built.

In this chapter, we begin by discussing the central role of play in time-limited MBT–C, before going on to describe a variety of techniques the therapist may use to assist the overall aims of the therapeutic work. All of the

http://dx.doi.org/10.1037/0000028-007
Mentalization-Based Treatment for Children: A Time-Limited Approach, by N. Midgley, K. Ensink, K. Lindqvist, N. Malberg, and N. Muller

techniques described here might be used with any children referred for time-limited MBT–C, but we have tried to describe them following a line of development, starting with those techniques that are more focused on helping children to establish the "building blocks" of the capacity to mentalize and moving on to those that focus more on the use of explicit mentalizing or that therapists can use when this capacity may break down. We end by describing some technical approaches in MBT–C to working with trauma and, in particular, helping children to develop a coherent narrative around traumatic experiences.

TIME-LIMITED MBT–C IS PLAY CENTERED

Play is a powerful medium, providing a way to explore relationships, to learn about the world of feelings, and to find one's own psychological voice as a child. Play is a form of social learning because all kinds of experiences in daily life are rehearsed, changed, and completed and, through these means, integrated in the behavior repertoire of a child.

- Play regulates negative affects and diminishes stress.
- Play helps metabolize major life events.
- Play integrates new information affectively and cognitively.
- Play offers a place to experiment with new behavior and new solutions.
- Play stimulates fantasy and fosters creativity.
- Play stimulates the development of empathy.
- Play stimulates the development of mentalizing. (Tessier, Normandin, Ensink, & Fonagy, 2016)

Winnicott (1971a) spoke of the need for the child's experience of a *transitional space*. It is this space that is metaphorically created in the process of the child's realization that she is separate yet connected, both physically and emotionally, from the parent. Play is one of the most fertile grounds for this process to take place, and this is one of the reasons play has always been such an essential component of psychodynamic and other play-based child therapies (Kegerreis & Midgley, 2014). As described in some of the early work on the development of the capacity to mentalize (Fonagy & Target, 1996b), when a child plays, she is learning to separate what she feels inside and how it is related, yet separate from what is in the external world. As Fonagy and Target (1998) noted, "the capacity to take a playful stance may be a critical step in the development of mentalization" (p. 108). However, an important ingredient in this process is the availability of an adult to help the child make sense of the experience by ensuring the child feels safe in the context of her explorations and by translating at times the world of emotions inside and outside.

When a child is playing, a range of interventions can be used with the aim of enhancing the child's awareness of mental states in himself and in others (Muñoz Specht, Ensink, Normandin, & Midgley, 2016). At the most basic level, this may involve simply *describing the play process*. The objective of this technique is to increase awareness and draw the child's attention to the way he plays during the therapy sessions. This is an active process in which the therapist summarizes and integrates all the information presented by the child during the play session (behaviors, affects, themes). For some children, this can help them to create an awareness of their own actions, or simply give them a sense that what they are doing can be seen and reflected on by someone else, that the therapist is curious about what they are doing. At a next level, the therapist may label and describe the child's actions in terms of mental states. This is done to highlight potentially problematic areas and helps to mentalize about the child's type of play, without overheating the emotional relationship by forcing the child to talk about painful or stressful situations that he is not ready to talk about.

Stimulating the Play Narrative

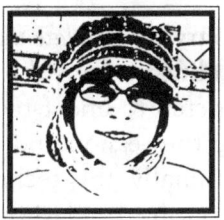

Twelve-year-old Ruth is inhibited and passive; she hardly speaks to the therapist. She sits quietly, appearing almost petrified, and seems unable to express interest or choose something to do. The therapist observes her uneasiness but decides not to focus attention on it; instead, he presents Ruth with potential ways of becoming more active and resolving her unease. He asks her if she wants to play or if she wants to make something, gently adding that she seems to find it hard to choose.

Although Ruth mostly only answers with her eyes, showing she understands what the therapist says, or replies with a simple yes or no, this time she quietly says she wants to make something. The therapist feels surprise and delight, but tones this down to attune to Ruth and not overwhelm her. The therapist believes that making something is a task that the child can do alone to affirm her agency; he has a sense that his role is to observe her agentic action and that this is the priority. He asks Ruth if she wants to draw or paint, or perhaps work with the clay. The therapist has the sense that he should offer some choices so that Ruth can have the experience of choosing and working with what is best for her, but not too many options, which could overwhelm her. Ruth answers that she wants to paint. He is pleased to hear what Ruth wants, expressing that he likes to know what she likes.

The therapist takes paper and the pots of paint out of the cupboard, asking Ruth if she wants to help and put the paint on the palette. Ruth does this, and the therapist comments and affirms Ruth's skillfulness in nicely putting little portions of paint on the palette all by herself. Then Ruth stands behind the easel with some white paper and indicates that she does not know what she should paint. The therapist tentatively asks her what comes to mind. Ruth says she doesn't know. The therapist is aware that this is a potentially important moment where Ruth is trying to take "authorship" of something, and is anxious that it should not end up in defeat and failure. At the same time, he wonders how he can best help and support Ruth and whether he should just simply focus on helping her tolerate the anxiety about finding what she wants to do and trust that something will emerge. He wonders to himself whether he should help out more actively as one might with a younger child, but without inadvertently sabotaging this moment when something new could potentially emerge by taking control too quickly and perhaps communicating to Ruth that he does not have confidence in her ability. He decides to turn it into a guessing game, saying that he's not sure what Ruth might like to paint—could it be a tree? her house? herself taking her dog for a walk? Ruth likes the third idea and seems to relax; she dips the paintbrush into the paint and starts with a surprisingly confident brushstroke.

At times it may be necessary for the therapist to try to *stimulate the play narrative* by asking questions with the aim of understanding the story the child is telling during the play. This technique is the first step to understanding the play context that the child is presenting during the session and helps the therapist make sense of what is going on. Additionally, this technique encourages the child to elaborate the stories presented during the play through gentle inquiry about the material presented and by asking for more details and descriptions. Such clarification and exploration, as Bateman and Fonagy (2012) pointed out, is not simply to establish facts; rather, it is to encourage the capacity to play with different ideas and perspectives.

In the preceding vignette, the therapist is actively trying to arrange the setting to facilitate Ruth's agency, supporting her and helping her feel secure and free to increasingly express herself. The therapist tries to draw her out from her passive position and help her discover that she can be more active—for example, in deciding what she wants to do—and also eventually take more of an active position in relationships by expressing what she wants to do rather than simply waiting and following others' lead. He thinks developmentally, mindful of how a parent may scaffold the agency of a young child by imagining what may be appropriate and giving options that the child might want to choose from. The therapist tries to be attuned to and affirm expressions of Ruth's agency and self, as well as her creativity, but he is careful not to inadvertently overwhelm Ruth so that she can feel the process belongs to her. He is guided by Ruth's reactions to adjust his reaction to the right level of intensity, thus scaffolding and encouraging Ruth. The therapist tries to create a safe space and a relationship in which Ruth experiences the therapist's benign interest in her internal world. At the same, time he is also able to wait and be "at the service" of Ruth's emerging self, not overwhelming her with his own enthusiasm because he is concerned that she should not subtly feel that she is doing this only to please the therapist. In sum, the therapist creates a potential space where Ruth can emerge and discover her more active, agentful self.

Mentalizing the Play

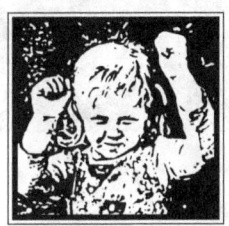

During a session toward the end of 6-year-old Anne's therapy, her interest shifts from somewhat repetitive play with cars to a set of figures in the sand tray (see Figure 6.1). The figures call either her or the therapist from the sand tray to consult them in different matters—for example, about how to take care of the wild animals that are moving into their playground. Through the play, the therapist and Anne explore what it is like for different animals to be together, what wishes and needs the animals may have, and how they think and feel. Some wild animals are still living nearby—a crocodile, a tiger, and a wolf—but they are in a cage and are no longer roaming freely or being a threat to the other animals. The therapist voices some worry about this through the figure of a small mouse: "Are you sure it's safe now, with the fence?" and Anne reassures her: "Yes, it's safe."

Anne arranges food for the animals to eat and explores the room to find things that can be used as food and cutlery. In different ways, she shows an emerging identification with a more caring role, showing her developing capacity for care, concern, and interest in the animals and their relationships. The therapist wonders whether the wild animals might sometimes want to come out of their cage and asks if they might not be feeling a bit trapped in there.

"I don't think they like the cage," says Anne, "but the mice would be scared if they were allowed out." The therapist accepts this but wonders whether they can find some way for both the wild animals and the farm animals to have some space to move about, while making sure the farm animals stay safe.

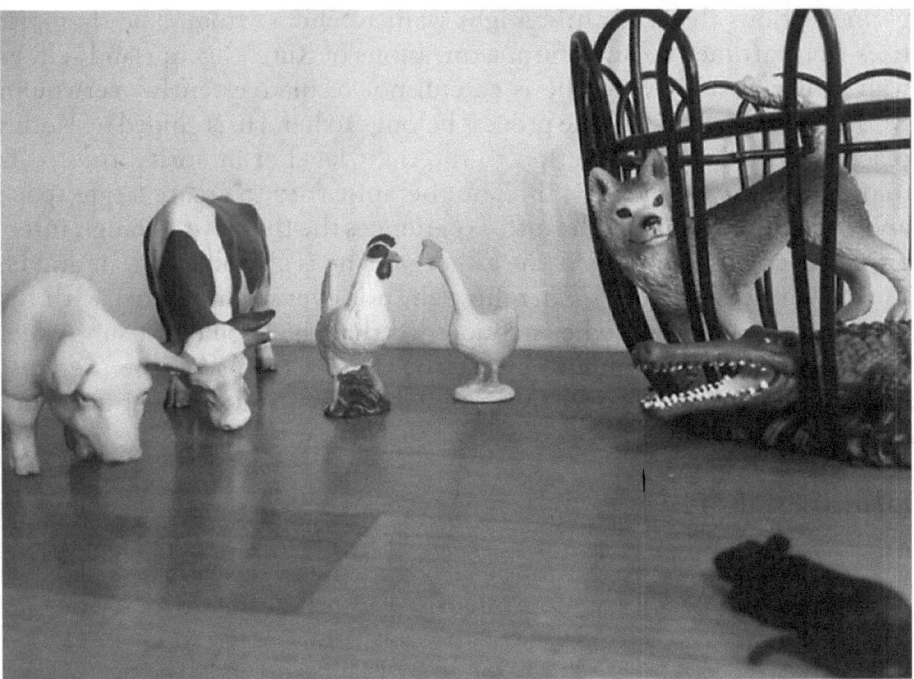

Figure 6.1. The animal figures in Anne's play.

Once a child is able to engage in symbolic play in an elaborated way, the therapist can focus on *mentalizing the narrative in the play context* (Muñoz Specht et al., 2016). This technique involves putting into words and clarifying and exploring the stories children present in their play and facilitating an elaboration of ideas and thoughts about these stories. Having an adult take on this function of commenting and putting into words the narrative of the play can be a powerful means of reflecting and consolidating the play ideas. This indicates that the relationship between child and therapist is one of coconstruction, sharing ideas, and listening to each other to explore and understand the story that best supports the child in what she wants to say. Sometimes this may involve *mentalizing characters and relationships in the play context* (Muñoz Specht et al., 2016). In doing this, the therapist is aiming to stimulate the mentalizing capacity of the child in a playful and unthreatening way by helping the child to think in terms of mental states about the play characters and their relationships during the play therapy session. This technique has to be used carefully, adopting a "wondering" approach so that the child does not feel dismissed or forced to accept the therapist's point of view about what characters in the play are thinking. But when done in a respectful way, it can help the therapist introduce more perspectives and the connections among thoughts, feelings, and behavior. This technique also seeks to help the child express her inner world and understand the inner world of others. Symbolic play provides a powerful medium for exploring, explicitly or implicitly, difficult feelings and expressing the way a child understands and deals with the world of relationships.

In Anne's play, we can observe her struggles between integrating good and bad feelings—angry crocodile feelings and mouse-like vulnerable feelings. Through the use of symbolic play, Anne's therapist is able to facilitate the expression and tolerance of both feelings and to gently explore the idea that different feelings might be able to "live together." By following the child and imagining, wondering, and putting into words the way the animals may be feeling, the therapist facilitates the emergence of richer and more flexible internal representations in the mind of the child and, most important, helps the child develop her capacity to play and use this as a way to communicate and express an inner source of creativity. She constructs and reconstructs an image of the different figures in her mind to help Anne think in mental-state terms by exploring what the animals may think, feel, or behave.

Valuing play implies that we are able to stay in touch with our own *playfulness as therapists*. Playfulness is an inner disposition to being open and experiencing freedom of thinking, feeling, and imagining; playfulness makes it possible to approach a topic or a problem from different perspectives and make contact with a child in a different way. It implies being open-minded and curious and letting go of standard ways of thinking and observing the content (Gluckers & Van Lier, 2011). Sometimes, holding back, letting the child experience an adult observing his play, and waiting for the story to emerge may be therapeutic. Playfulness is a way of being free and creative, and although the play in MBT–C should mostly be child-led, the therapist can introduce playful elements that might help the child become freer or less inhibited. Child therapists sometimes worry if they are "just playing" (Hurry, 1998) or if they are introducing their own ideas into a play situation; but play can be therapeutic in and of itself, and it is for that reason that Barish (2009) encouraged those working with children to "relax with child patients—to be animated and playful, at times even silly" (p. 83). However, when therapists find themselves introducing elements into the play, a self-reflexive process in which the therapist reflects on the work after the session may be particularly important. The therapist may reflect on whether she contributed something meaningful by introducing a play theme or character to help the child elaborate a central issue, for example. This is usually consciously planned but may also be spontaneous. Sometimes the therapist may be modeling, at an appropriate moment, that playfulness, silliness, and fun are allowed and can be enjoyed.

Thus, we suggest that therapists practice a degree of self-monitoring. This may be especially important if they are left with a sense of discomfort about their interventions after a session or when they notice that they became more active than usual or introduced new themes, rather than following the child's themes.

When Children Cannot Engage in Symbolic Play

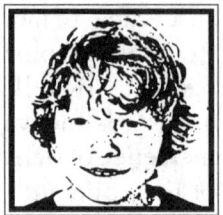 John, who is 8 years old, comes in with an angry expression. He doesn't want, or isn't able, to tell the therapist what happened that made him so angry. In previous sessions, he always seemed to calm down while playing with clay, so the therapist asks him if he wants to use the clay, which John accepts. When the therapist and John both have a piece of clay, the therapist asks John if he wants to smash the clay on the table so it's easier to handle. Her idea (although she doesn't say this to him) is that it might help John direct his anger into throwing the clay, communicating to him in an implicit way that his anger is seen and that it is OK, as well as signaling to him that she is available and he is allowed to find a way to express some of his feelings with her.

John sighs deeply, with a mixture of despair and relief, and looks to the therapist when he smashes the clay with all his force, seeming to double-check that he is not scaring her and whether expressing his anger in this way is acceptable to her. Going one step further, in response to the pleasure John seems to have in throwing the clay, the therapist suggests that he should climb up onto the table and smash the clay onto the ground from up high. John first thinks the therapist is joking, but when he sees her smile, he looks excited and climbs up onto the table. The therapist explains that this is not something they would usually do, but she has the impression John really needs to smash his clay from a big distance today.

John is completely focused and puts all his strength into throwing the clay. When the clay hits the ground, it makes a big noise, like a fart. John laughs out loud. The therapist laughs with him. John's face starts relaxing, and he seems open and connected with the therapist. She asks him who he would like to have lying on the floor where he is throwing his clay. John responds by connecting his feelings to a frustrating incident that happened at school, saying, "Luke teased me the whole day and called me a pig, and I tried not to fight, but in the end I did and my teacher was angry with me and not with Luke and that was so mean!"

The therapist, happy that John could tell her about his emotions, gives him the clay again and says, "Well, then, it sounds like he deserves this clay. Do you feel like giving it all you've got?"

John throws again and again and is standing on the table doing a monkey drum on his chest, feeling strong, feeling in control, and looking really pleased.

The therapist says, "Sometimes it's just so great to let it all out when you know you can't hurt anyone or get into trouble. Those situations are so frustrating when these guys set you up and provoke you, and you know they want to get you into trouble. You try your best, but in the end, they walk away while you get into trouble."

John nods and seems to relax. He starts cleaning up the mess and then adds thoughtfully, "Well, I thought you'd be proud of me—I controlled myself and only pushed him, when I actually felt like punching him right in the face!"

Of course not all children who are referred to therapy are able to make use of symbolic play. As children get older, they become less inclined to play but may be able to use drawing and clay. For older children, board games can be used to address issues around rules and losing, but for some children, physical games, such as playing with a hockey puck and sticks, can be useful to practice control and care. This provides a therapeutic opportunity to think about how to keep everyone safe, because either the therapist or the child may get hurt if the play becomes too rough. When a child cannot or will not participate in pretend play, activities that involve the body and movement may be helpful. Typical activities can include playing with balls (e.g., tossing balls back and forth), sword fighting, playing music together, or playing in a gym.

In the preceding vignette, the therapist is aware that John has been struggling with his anger and that he is desperately afraid he will be rejected if he expresses anger. He has had few opportunities to have anger normalized by understanding that we all feel angry sometimes and that anger can be important for overcoming obstacles, coping when someone has hurt us, or protecting ourselves. However, therapists need to learn to use it effectively, rather than be blinded or controlled by it. Furthermore, John has probably had few, if any, opportunities to talk freely about how angry he feels and have this accepted and tolerated. The therapist has the sense that it is important for John to learn that angry feelings are normal and can be accepted and validated so that he can learn to be less afraid of anger and begin to see it as something normal that can be controlled. In suggesting that John throw the clay at the floor, the therapist communicates that she is not afraid of his anger and invites John to express it in the room with her. She gives him permission to express his physical anger and frustration in a somewhat wild, but also controlled, way. The therapist is engaging with him (and even encouraging him) in this activity as a means of helping him express the feelings he is so afraid of and thinks are forbidden and unacceptable, so that they can become less frightening and dangerous. Through this process, the therapist communicates that she is not afraid of John's feelings even when they are "big, angry feelings," that they can be expressed without hurting others, and that it is human to feel this way. She hopes that in this way, he might begin to feel less afraid and have a sense that his feelings can be tolerated, accepted, and thought about, paving the way for self-acceptance and self-regulation.

The use of clay or a sand tray can also help establish contact with children who present as inhibited or unwilling. All these activities have in common that they do not demand any fine motor skills but also can be used to play with rhythm, force, and rituals. When a ball is thrown, the therapist may illustrate (mirror) with a sound the force and the course of the ball. When playing music together, the therapist can lead the way in experimenting with volume, rhythm, and tempo. Activities that stimulate the senses may be good for children not yet able to play symbolically (e.g., encouraging them to feel how the sand, water, clay, or paint feels in their hands).

Ensuring That Interventions Are Adapted to the Right Level for the Child

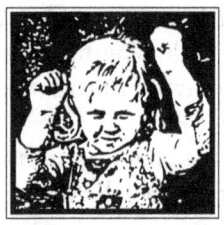 It is the 10th session, and Anne is playing with the dolls and the animals at the table, elaborating a theme that has been central throughout therapy. She returns to a game that she has played before, in which the lion cub runs away from the therapist's doll but then suddenly turns round and hits it. The therapist, mindful that they are coming toward the end of their 12 sessions, wonders aloud whether today the lion cub is unsure if she likes the doll or is angry with her. Anne tells her to shut up and play. The therapist notices Anne's agitation but continues to explore why the lion club may be feeling grumpy like this today. Anne gets increasingly frustrated and eventually throws the lion cub into the corner of the room and screams at the therapist, "I hate you!" Before the therapist can do anything, Anne runs to the door and runs crying back to the waiting room.

In previous chapters, we spoke about the importance of not expecting children to be able to mentalize explicitly when they are in a heightened emotional state that may have led their mentalizing capacity to go "offline."

Verheugt-Pleiter (2008b) referred to this as "recognizing the child's level of mental functioning and meeting it at the same level" (p. 57), acknowledging that therapists sometimes have a tendency to speak at a level that is too abstract, assuming, for example, that a child may be able to be curious about why the therapist may have said something when at that moment the child is certain he has said it to hurt her.

Given that high arousal is often a trigger for a breakdown in mentalizing, even in children who have developed some capacity to reflect on mental states, in the therapy room with a child, the therapist must be continually judging the "emotional temperature" and trying to ensure that her interventions meet the child at the right level. When we sometimes get this wrong, as we inevitably will, all we can do is acknowledge our mistake and try to recover. For example, in the preceding vignette, Anne's therapist is mindful that their short-term intervention is coming to an end, and before beginning the session, she had gone back to remind herself what the agreed focus had been for the therapy: "Getting to know and taking care of the wild animals and the wild emotions." But in her own anxiety about ensuring that she and Anne were on track with the therapy, she lost sight of Anne's emotional state in the room, inviting her to explicitly mentalize about the lion cub ("I wonder why she may be feeling like this today?") when Anne was in an agitated state (at this stage, we can only guess why), which makes this kind of controlled, reflective activity impossible. This is a common mistake among novice (and more experienced) MBT–C therapists, who may ask questions that invite explicit mentalizing (e.g., "How do you think your mum felt when you did that?" "Why are you feeling like that now?") when the child is in an emotional state in which their capacity to mentalize is "offline."

In thinking about "which intervention when?" Bateman and Fonagy (2006), in the context of MBT for adults, introduced the idea of a spectrum of interventions, ranged according to their complexity, as well as their depth and emotional intensity. These range from offering empathy and support, which they described as being "the simplest most superficial and least intensive, to mentalizing the relationship, as the most complex and, for the most part, the most emotionally intensive" (p. 111). In a similar way, Jacobsen, Ha, and Sharp (2015), describing their work with children in foster care, talked about a "mentalizing staircase," from being supportive and empathic when there are high levels of emotional intensity in the room, to reflecting on the minds of self and other when the child is calmer. As Taylor (2012) put it, "high arousal states are responded to by simple mentalizing efforts such as support and empathy; low arousal states by high mentalizing states such as exploring and interpreting thinking" (p. 166). As therapists, we are almost certain to get this wrong at times and pitch things at the wrong level for a child at certain moments. This is inevitable, but the important thing is to try to recognize when we do this, apologize, and try again. When in doubt, it is always best to fall back on the fundamental aspects of the mentalizing stance set out in Chapter 4, including being curious ("Wow, what did I just do there?"), empathic ("I can see you got really upset when I asked you what it was like for your mom when you did that."), and then, in time, try to understand the misunderstanding ("Now that things are calmer, can we just go back and see what happened?").

Building Foundations to Support Mentalizing

As we have argued previously, regulation of attention and affect facilitates mentalizing, and this is necessary to be able to keep in mind the thoughts and feelings of oneself and others and then use this ability interpersonally. Many school-age children referred to psychological services have an underdeveloped capacity for this or tend to easily lose this capacity. When children are easily affectively dysregulated, show impulsivity, or have little capacity to think about themselves and relationships in mental-state terms, it can be therapeutic to focus on building these foundations that support mentalizing by working on capacities for basic self-regulation, attention control, and affect regulation. With some children, this will be the focus for much of the therapeutic work; with others, it may be possible to work simultaneously with their more explicit mentalizing skills, including more controlled, reflective exploration of the mental states of self and other. The therapeutic work is always guided by the therapist's assessment of the child's capacity for regulation and mentalization, both globally and at a moment-by-moment level, and may include the following:

- stimulating contact by working on attunement and joint attention,
- mirroring and contingent coordination,
- creating rhythm and patterns in interactions,
- enhancing attention control and self-awareness by naming and describing what is happening in the here and now,
- promoting intentionality by linking behavior to effects in the external world,
- regulating affects by exaggerating or slowing down,
- regulating attention and affects by setting and playing with limits,
- clarifying and naming feeling states, and
- using games or activities.

Attunement, Mirroring, and Contingent Coordination

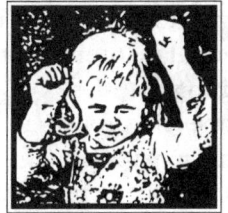 In a session with her MBT–C therapist, Anne uses swords and hits them against each other. The therapist imitates the sound by saying, "bam, bam, bam!" Anne laughs and hits hard. The therapist comments that Anne hits hard, and she makes loud noises! Anne then finds a kettle and wants go and get water for it. She wants to do it herself. She fills the kettle to the brim. The therapist notes that it's very full and wonders if maybe they need to pour some out. Anne says "No!" and insists that she will walk carefully. She does this, and the therapist comments that she is indeed very strong and can walk very carefully. Then Anne finds a toy syringe from a doctor's kit, sucks water into the syringe, and wants to spray it out. When she wants to spray water in the doll's pram, the therapist says no, but Anne sprays some water there anyway.

The therapist says, "You know what, you can spray in the sand tray; you see here are two sand trays!"

Anne wants to spray in the tray with dry sand, but the therapist suggests that she sprays in the tray with the wet sand, and Anne follows her directions.

Anne and the therapist repeat this over and over again: Anne sucks water into the syringe (which is really small) and the therapist tells her when it's full (because it's difficult to see) and then Anne sprays it in the sand. Sometimes she pushes so hard that she sprays water on the toys on the shelves, and she laughs happily. The therapist makes sound effects when Anne pulls the syringe apart to be able to fill it with water (it makes a popping sound, and the therapist says "POP!"). Anne laughs at it the first time, and then they say it together as she pulls it apart and when she sprays the water. Anne and the therapist walk between the table with the water and the sand tray over and over again. When Anne sprays all over the shelf with the toys, the therapist smiles and comments that it was very far to reach the right place.

Children who are chaotic and disorganized or who don't seem to be grounded in their bodies may not have developed the foundations that can help to support mentalizing. At times, they may seem unaware of what they are doing and why, and it can be challenging for the therapist to make contact. There is also a risk of turning into a "police officer," making sure that nothing in the room gets damaged. Sometimes the first step has to do with making contact with the child, even if for fleeting moments, to let the child know that the session is a safe place and to try to increase the child's attention to aspects of her own experience. The *therapist's contingent coordination with the child*, drawing on nonverbal modalities such as making a soothing sound with a soft tone of voice or a facial expression full of compassion, can be important therapeutic interventions. Such interventions can help these children to attend to and process information and modulate their emotions, before opening the door to developing other mentalizing abilities.

With children like Anne, much of the therapeutic process may be about "*creating patterns of being together* rather than only what is actually said" (Verheugt-Pleiter, 2008a, p. 113, emphasis added). It is about trying to create rhythm, predictability, joint attention, and a feeling of togetherness. In the session with Anne just described, the therapist tries to imitate, synchronize, and make contact at a nonverbal level. At the same time, he is trying to make Anne more aware of her own body and its force. The therapist is trying to turn the child's inward and enhance self-awareness. This can be done, for example, by *naming and describing what's happening in the here and now*, such as physical states and actions (*"You hit hard! You are using all your force! Bam, bam, bam!"*). This work has many elements of nonverbal attunement (mirroring). The focus is on what Anne is doing, and the therapist is joining her in the play. What Anne does (banging swords, pouring water, throwing pucks) and how the therapist reacts can also be seen as *introducing some affect regulation*—becoming aware that one's own expressions and behaviors can be modulated, that Anne can regulate and modulate things she does and thus also modulate the effect of her behavior on the external world. The therapist links the child's behavior ("you hit hard") with the effect in the external world ("there's a loud noise"). This is the beginning of working on an implicit concept of intentional behavior. At the same time, the therapist herself is managing her own arousal level because she is worried that the play could get out of hand. In doing this, she is also trying to regulate the emotional level of the child, in an implicit and playful way, and slowly but surely introducing more rules and limits. The therapist gently introduces the idea of limits in a flexible way, not being punitive when Anne does not comply but reiterating and directing where a good place is to squirt the water until Anne is able to comply. This is much as one might do with a younger child.

Setting and playing with limits in the therapy room develops and practices regulatory abilities in several ways. When Anne plays at home or school, it often ends in chaos and destruction. At the beginning of therapy, she often impulsively poured liters of water on the floor in the therapy room, then worried about the mess she had made. The therapist wanted to help Anne gain a sense that she could play without things getting out control. She also regulates the emotional excitement, trying to create awareness in Anne of what she's doing, implying that she has a choice. For many boisterous children like Anne who come for treatment, developing the capacity to accept limits or develop internal control is a major challenge, and they often get punished and rejected at school and elsewhere unless they are able to develop such control. However, these children often get little help in doing so, setting off a negative spiral, with implications for their self-esteem. Practicing these kinds of negotiations and trying to regulate affects related to them can be an important aspect of the therapeutic work and can be done playfully.

The therapist is also actively creating opportunities to help Anne think about the situations that pose difficulties using a "school" installed in the corner of the sand tray. The two of them play with the idea, saying that sometimes it is fine to express oneself freely, but at other times and in other environments, it is important to learn to follow the rules even when it is hard to do so. Anne seems to respond and engage with this practice with the therapist. Therapists may feel ambivalent about engaging in this type of playful practicing and be concerned that it is not traditional play therapy. However, practicing and elaborating in play the situations in which the child gets stuck can be valuable in helping her elaborate, see, and think about these difficulties creatively. It implies that the therapist has done a mental microanalysis in which the problem is broken down and each step in the sequence of events is imagined until the problem can be clearly pictured, as in a mental video. The therapist can ask the child, "Is this what happens?" or "Show me what happens now," and they can physically walk through the sequence—for example, from arriving at school, hanging up their coats. They may go on to eat their pretend snack, up to the moment when the bully approaches and provokes or teases the child, until she snaps and gets sent off to the principal's office. As they go through each part, it may be possible to explore mental states in the self and other by asking questions such as, "So what was going on for you right then?" or "What do you think was in her mind when she said that?" With some children, this can also be done by creating a cartoon series together.

Using play in this way can be an important stepping-stone toward more sophisticated play activity. Later on, as Anne's play changed and became more symbolic, she started playing more with the tiger and farm animals, the therapist was able to use this creatively. For example, they could "take the tiger to school" together or teach the tiger some deep-breathing exercises when he started having roaring feelings and wanted to bite. Together they could write a little comic book manual especially for tigers who want to start school but are afraid that they might bite someone, addressing step by step each of the difficulties that a little tiger is likely to face at school and his strategies to overcome these difficulties.

As part of this marked mirroring process, as described in Chapter 1 in the context of parent–child interactions, the therapist may make use of *ostensive cues*. This might involve calling attention to what the therapist is about to communicate (e.g., by making direct eye contact with the child while calling the child by name or tilting the head toward the child and changing the intonation of her voice slightly). For a traumatized child, it may be important *not* to offer direct eye contact but to call the child's name and talk with her without activating a fight-or-flight response; in some cases, it can be helpful for the child to have an activity that she can focus on so that the intensity of the relationship is somewhat hidden as she pays attention to the joint activity and slowly eases into the relationship.

In communicating in this way, the therapist's expression of emotion can be marked by modifying (e.g., exaggerating or slowing down) the display of the child's affect, such that the therapist's emotional expression resembles but regulates the child's emotion simultaneously. The idea is not that the therapist should be perfectly accurate every time that she comments on what might be going on for the child but that the child senses that the therapist is interested in her experience, able to follow and stay in emotional contact with her and that she experiences the therapist's genuine interest in her mind.

At times, this process happens at a nonverbal level, especially for children who have little emotional vocabulary that could help them to describe their internal states. The therapist often has to be imaginative and resourceful to find a way to reach and engage children in such states. This is particularly important when working with children whose aggression easily gets out of control and whose apparent incapacity to play may represent a safety measure to protect themselves and others from the strength of their angry feelings and their perception of themselves as unable to manage these feelings. It can be equally important when children have faced almost unspeakable trauma and loss and can gradually help them build up an experience of, and attention to, subjective states: "This is me, I can have intentions, wishes, feelings, and thoughts." The child may also become more curious about the other: "There is someone out there who seems to be interested in me and wants to be in contact with me."

Clarifying and Naming Feeling States

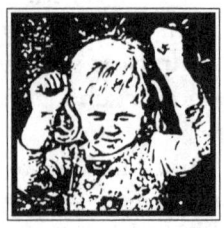 During an early session the therapist feels that Anne needs help developing an emotional vocabulary, so she decides to bring in a specific activity. She shows Anne a card with a picture of a boy peeking out from behind a sofa (see Figure 6.2) and asks her to tell a little story. "Ooooh, there is a child hiding behind the couch," says Anne. The therapist encourages her to elaborate his story further, to find out why he is sitting there, and what he is feeling.

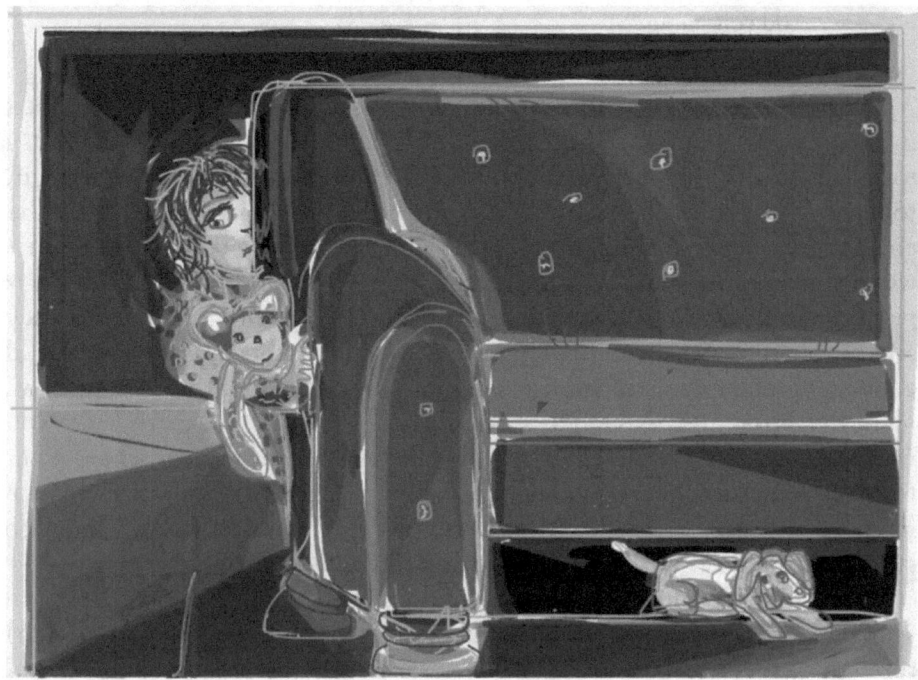

Figure 6.2. The drawing of a child peeking out from behind the sofa from work with Anne. Drawing by Ruth Zuilhof, The Hague, The Netherlands.

Anne guesses that he is hiding, but says she can't say what the boy might be feeling. "Do you think maybe he is afraid, or sad or playing a trick on someone by hiding?" asks the therapist.

Although Anne first says she doesn't know, with the therapist's encouragement to look at the boy's face, she guesses that the boy is sad, adding, "Yes, he has a sad look in his eyes."

The therapist is impressed with this comment, and Anne then starts talking about a time when she felt sad, when she was separated from her mother in an amusement park. With the therapist's encouragement, she gives a detailed account of what happened. The therapist wonders what she felt when she couldn't find her mother, and Anne tells her that it was her own fault—"Because I wanted to play in the playground and wanted to stay there."

The therapist shows sympathy with how Anne felt. "Yes and then I had to cry out loud and a lady asked me what happened, and I said 'I don't know where my mommy is' and then we started to look for my mom and then we saw her." The therapist asks whether Anne remembers how she felt when she saw her mother's face, and she tells her she was happy.

"And your mom?"

"She was happy too, but also a little angry," she replies.

On the basis of the slow process of contingent coordination described in the previous section, the therapist in MBT–C can gradually begin to try to make connections between action and emotions and clarify and begin to *name feeling states*. This might begin with the therapist simply asking the child to tell her what she wants (e.g., saying "Today, maybe you can tell me when you are thirsty and which toys you feel like playing with"). The therapist thus scaffolds the development of the child's capacity to express agency and her feelings and to ask for what she needs in relationships. When a child expresses preferences and starts asking for particular toys, the therapist can mark this by comments such as, "Look at you—you know exactly what you want!" She can also help the child become aware that she can express her feelings, sometimes through play (e.g., when playing with dolls, say, "Maybe if the baby learns to *say* she feels scared of the dark, then we will know to switch the light on in the hall so she doesn't have to cry?").

For some children it can be helpful for the therapist to bring in more structured ways of helping the child name feelings. Asen and Fonagy (2012a) referred to these as *mentalization-enhancement activities* and gave the example of a "Guess Your Feelings" game that can be used in a family session. Alternatively, one can use picture books or drawings, as the therapist did with Anne when she used picture cards to initiate a conversation about feelings. Anne did not start talking about feelings spontaneously, but when the therapist gave some suggestions, she was able to make a good guess about the emotions of the boy behind the couch. She could also, when prompted by the therapist, link the way the boy in the picture looks to emotions, indicating that she had some understanding of emotional expressions. She was then able to tell the therapist about an incident when she felt sad. The therapist noticed Anne's emotional involvement when she told the story. She expressed sadness and fear when talking, and she had a smile on her face when she came to the end of the story; she even showed awareness of how someone could hold two different feelings simultaneously. When the therapist reacted and commented on the story, she was deliberately emotionally expressive as well.

Using pictures like that in Figure 6.2 may help children talk about feelings, especially those children who may need more scaffolding to name emotions. With many children, it is possible to ask them to make up a little story about what is happening in the picture. With Anne, however, the therapist got the impression that Anne did not seem open to imagining about the characters in the picture (only answering with very short sentences or saying "I don't know" when being asked to guess what happened in the picture). So the therapist decided to ask directly about a story from Anne's real life; Anne responded more enthusiastically.

For other children, the play can be an opportunity to *notice and name feeling states*.

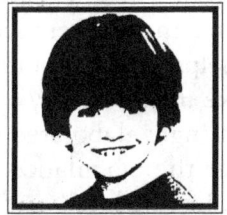

In one of the early sessions, Mohammed, age 7, plays with a police car and a doll. He is banging the doll and the car on the table, shouting loudly. When the therapist speaks, he ignores her. He keeps banging the doll and the car, until the therapist touches his arm gently and tries to find his eyes to make sure there is some contact. "There is a lot of banging and screaming. It looks like someone may be getting hurt! Who is screaming so loudly?" she asks.

"I am," Mohammed says.

The therapist then comments, staying in the play, "Are you OK, or are you hurt? Are you afraid? Do you need some help there?"

"Yes," Mohammed says with a sigh, looking at his therapist for a split second.

She makes sure she is mirroring the boy's expression. "Show me what happened," the therapist says in an exaggerated, slow tone of voice, as she looks at the doll and the car in Mohammed's hands as he bashes them together and screams. She adds, "Hmm . . . all that noise, with lots of people screaming and shouting. That sounds very confusing and scary" (showing with her face and bringing her hands to cover her ears).

Mohammed smiles slightly and seems to be considering what to do next. The therapist comments on this: "Big feelings inside, big sounds outside?"

Mohammed smiles, gets up, and runs around the room and then sits back down and seems ready to start playing again.

The therapist asks, "I wonder what is happening next? What are the police doing? Do we need to call an ambulance?"

In this example, the therapist notices that Mohammed is becoming dysregulated, as the play appears to be evoking some of the strong feelings linked to the car crash he experienced in real life. She notices that there is a feeling of being out of contact with Mohammed, who does not seem to be "in the room" and seems unaware of how loudly he is screaming. He seems lost in repetitive traumatic play in which he is reliving the trauma rather than mentally processing and metabolizing it by elaborating the experience in the play. Mohammed seems to dissociate as the play stirs up powerful trauma-related feelings in him. In using his name and touching him gently on the arm, the therapist brings Mohammed back into the room and interrupts the dissociative process, so that he can benefit from the process of representing the trauma and developing semantic discourse about it with the scaffolding of the therapist's verbal commentary on his play, rather than simply reliving the most traumatic affects. She chooses to not specifically name the feelings of fear at this point because she is not sure whether he is ready and is concerned that he will stop playing; but at a future point when he plays this trauma-related scene again, she will talk about him having felt very scared. Through her verbal commentary on his play, she helps him elaborate the traumatic experience and put it into words and make it into a story with a beginning, a middle, and an end that can be increasingly elaborated until it contains all the essential elements (e.g., whether the ambulance took anyone to hospital) so that Mohammed is not stuck just with reliving only the most traumatic moment of the crash and the unbearable affects at that moment.

Working With Explicit Mentalizing and Breakdowns in Mentalizing

In Chapter 2, we described how at times the capacity for mentalizing, even when it has been established in the child, can break down, either on a temporary or more chronic basis. Often this may take the form of a switch away from more controlled, explicit mentalizing toward a nonmentalizing mode of functioning, usually in the context of heightened emotional states of stress or arousal. As Zevalkink, Verheugt-Pleiter, and Fonagy (2012) put it,

> What is therapeutic in MBT–C is 1) the identification of the loss on mentalizing as it occurs and 2) not allowing the child to continue in a non-mentalizing mode for too long but confronting non-mentalizing and replacing it with a more adaptive mode of thinking about self and others in a social (attachment) context. (p. 143)

In this section, we describe some of the techniques that the therapist can draw on to support this process, which may include the following:

- offering support and empathy in the face of dysregulation and/or mentalizing breakdowns;
- stop, rewind, and explore;
- looking for and validating mental states, such as thoughts, feelings, wishes, and intentions, in stories and play;
- enhancing perspective-taking and differentiation between self and others by mentalizing relationships, inside and outside therapy; and
- creating mentalizing narratives around difficult life experiences or traumatic events.

Offering Empathy and Support in the Face of Mentalizing Breakdowns

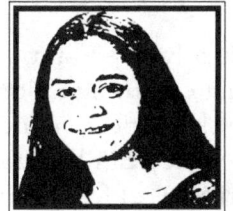 Liza, 11 years old, comes to the session saying she had an accident this morning, when she fell over. No one saw it, but an ambulance came; Liza explains, "Because I was OK, I didn't need an ambulance, so I just sent them back to the hospital."

The therapist had wondered before how to handle moments in which Liza told something that clearly wasn't true, without a sense of connectedness with her inner feelings in the way she told them or her way of dealing with reality. The therapist noticed that it felt difficult to show real empathy for Liza at these moments, but this time she decides to try to validate Liza's feelings by saying, "You must have been very startled. Gosh, it's good of you to tell me."

When that doesn't appear to have any impact, the therapist decides to overexaggerate her response and makes a joke about the ambulance, saying, "And the ambulance and the police and the fire squad all came to rescue you."

Liza and the therapist laugh together, and Liza says, "Well, I really thought the ambulance would have to come because I really felt bad."

This feels much more genuine, and the therapist can react in a more real way by responding empathically: "Yes, I can imagine you must have thought it was really serious because it felt so painful. Sometimes it seems your feeling is so big, you make your story a little bigger too, perhaps?"

Liza grins, and it feels as if there is a moment of connection.

In this vignette, Liza appears to have arrived at the session after having had some kind of fall that morning, which is likely to have activated her attachment needs. However, as a child with a more avoidant attachment style, she minimized these needs presented the situation in an overly cognitive way, with her account lacking in emotional resonance. She then went off into a flight of fantasy, in which reality and pretending became confused. The therapist noticed how this seemed to be played out in the way the two of them interacted in the session, with the therapist herself feeling rather distant and uninvolved. Noticing this in herself, she was able to think how Liza was operating in pretend mode and that, rather than engage with her at a cognitive level (e.g., "So why do you think the ambulance came all the way out and then just went straight back?"), she was able to *validate the feeling* behind the story to try to bring Liza's mentalizing capacity back online. This did not happen at first, so the therapist introduced some humor into the situation. Although it can be a little risky to challenge a child in the way that the therapist did here, the humor can allow a more real contact, which in this case was followed up by a recognition of the real feelings that the child was experiencing.

Supportive and empathic interventions are particularly important during moments when the child seems emotionally dysregulated; the aim is to help regulate the heightened or (as in this case) diminished affective arousal. Such interventions have an additional importance: They can help reduce a child's level of epistemic mistrust. Repeated experiences of feeling understood and supported in this way can lead a child to gradually have a sense that it may be safe to trust and therefore to begin to take on board what the other is offering.

Stop and Rewind

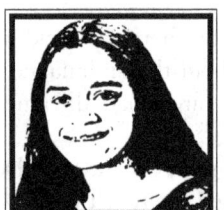 Liza is playing cards in her session. During the game, she suddenly realizes that the therapist is applying a rule, which she had forgotten to apply earlier, and in a firm tone that is unusual given her generally timid demeanor, Liza says, "Wait, I didn't do that when it was my turn!"

With this the atmosphere of being close and complicit in playing a game together changes immediately, and Liza throws her pieces onto the table. Responding to this change, the therapist comments, "Can we just stop for a moment? What just happened there? One moment we were playing together, and suddenly it feels tense."

Liza doesn't reply, but the emotional temperature in the room seems to have settled again.

"Can we just go back and think what happened there?" the therapist asks again, and this time Liza nods.

After retracing what had happened step by step, the therapist suddenly hits on an idea, and asks, "Did you maybe think I made you miss out on purpose?"

Liza nods again, and says yes, that was exactly what she felt. The therapist is able to thank her for explaining this because now she can understand why Liza got so upset with her. "It must feel awful to think I tricked you on purpose," she says, with feeling.

At this point, Liza says they should carry on with the game, and they do. A little while later, while still playing, the therapist asks, "Liza, I'm just wondering, do you think there's any other reasons I might have not reminded you about the rule?"

Liza shrugs her shoulders, and says, "Maybe you just forgot?"

"Yes, I think you're right," says her therapist, "at least as far as I know. I certainly didn't mean to do it, but I'm sorry I did."

Later they come back to this again, and the therapist is able to talk to Liza about whether this kind of thing happens elsewhere in her life and how what happened here might link to what happens in her home or at school, when she feels like a fool when others know rules but don't tell her. They then use it to their advantage to gain things she worked hard for, so she feels tricked and defeated, as if she will never know all the rules and will always lose.

Once the therapist has seen that a child's mentalizing has broken down, and offered the kind of supportive and empathic response that can help to bring the capacity back online, it is possible to work together to explore and learn from such experiences, making use of more, reflective thinking. To do this, it can often be helpful to slow things down, using a technique that Bateman and Fonagy (2012) referred to as *stop and rewind*. The purpose of using this strategy, they wrote, is "to reinstate mentalizing when it has been lost or to promote its continuation in the furtherance of the overall goal of therapy, which is . . . to encourage the formation of a robust and flexible mentalizing capacity that is not prone to sudden collapse in the face of emotional stress" (p. 132). By doing so, the therapist actively interrupts the nonmentalizing interaction and slows things down before asking questions with the aim of reconstructing the events that led to the mentalizing breakdown.

In the preceding example, it may not have been helpful for the therapist to explain at first, "Well, of course I didn't do it on purpose. I am here to help you." Although that may be true, it would assume that Liza had the capacity to be curious about what was in the mind of the other and to consider a different perspective. The child, in psychic equivalence mode at this time, is convinced that what she thinks is the truth, and nothing but the truth. What is helpful for Liza is that her therapist shows empathy and acknowledges the reality of her internal reality and experience ("That must feel awful to think I tricked you on purpose."). In this way, Liza feels acknowledged in her experience, and trust is beginning to be established. As soon as the therapist notices that the emotional temperature had changed in the room, she stops the play and tries to help Liza to begin self-observing and thinking about what happened between the two of them. Later in the session, they explore together how this happens in other relationships as well.

The stop, rewind, and explore process is a powerful tool to address mentalizing breakdowns. In this way, the therapist is facilitating a process of perspective-taking by providing possible hypothesis, displaying curiosity about what Liza feels and what she thinks others feel or think, and at times introducing different possibilities. Talking about a situation in the here and now can help generate new representations about feelings from situations outside therapy as well.

Mentalizing the Relationship

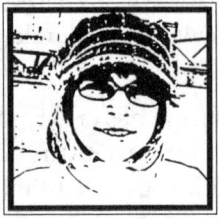 Ruth sits in the corner of the room. As she plays with the big stuffed bear, she ignores her therapist completely. When the silence continues, the therapist wonders out loud that there are "no words in the room today" and wonders what could be going on. Ruth responds by pretending to be sleeping for a while and complains out loud: "This is soooo boring."

The therapist looks confused, and with a somewhat exaggerated facial expression says, "Hmm, that's so confusing."

"What?" Ruth asks.

"Well," the therapist replies, "last week we had such a lot of fun together playing cards, and then when it was time to go, you seemed grumpy . . . I wonder if you might still be grumpy because we had to stop our fun."

Ruth replies: "Shut up! You just don't get it!"

The therapist asks her if they can wind things back so he can understand what he got wrong. Ruth is hesitant at first, but after a while she says that she realized after the last session that her therapist only plays with her because he's paid to do so. "What makes you think that?" asks the therapist, and Ruth says that she noticed the therapist looking at his watch several times before ending the last session.

Ruth and her therapist talk this through for some time, with the therapist trying to understand why Ruth interpreted his behavior this way. The therapist says he understands that it is painful to feel someone you enjoy being with seems more concerned about the time, and perhaps this is what makes Ruth hesitant to engage today. Ruth shrugs her shoulders, but her attitude seems to have softened, so the therapist continues and acknowledges that he was anxious about the time as the last session ended, but from his side, it was because he could see Ruth was enjoying it and wanted to make sure that he didn't interrupt things too abruptly. Ruth remains somewhat unconvinced, but she does begin to see that there may be other reasons why her therapist looked at his watch and that it was probably not because he wanted to get rid of her. She starts to bounce the bear that was on her lap around the room and then throws it at the therapist, who replies, "Is that an invitation not to lose more of our time and just get the fun going?"

Ruth smiles, "Shut up and just play! Let's do some coloring."

The therapist asks what is special about coloring, and Ruth replies, "So I can calm down. . . . I hate it that the time goes so fast in here and the sessions are so short. Let's play and not waste more time."

Bateman and Fonagy (2012) explained that the aim of mentalizing the relationship is to

focus the patient's attention on another mind, the mind of a therapist, and to assist the patient in the task of contrasting their own perception of themselves with how they are perceived by another, and thought about differently by different minds. (p. 139)

Although bearing some similarity to the work of transference interpretation, the aim is not so much to provide insight into repetitive patterns of relating but rather to give further opportunity to experience how recovering the capacity to mentalize can help interpersonal relationships.

In Ruth's case, the experiences of losing people and of wanting more from grown-ups begins to show in the treatment only a few weeks after beginning therapy. She seems to enjoy her sessions, but this seems to activate the attachment system, and suddenly she is reminded of the pain of loss and also her feeling that she always gets the "short end of the stick." By staying with what the child brings in the here and now to the session, the therapist once again uses a process of stop and rewind, but he goes beyond this to try to *mentalize the relationship*. When the initial supportive and empathic response reduces the high arousal level and Ruth's affect is better regulated, the therapist invites some *explicit mentalizing*, encouraging Ruth to think about other possible reasons the therapist had been checking his watch. At a certain stage, he shares his own, different perspective on why he may have been doing that. Through this slow process, Ruth is able to recover her capacity to mentalize and responds to the therapist's attempts to invite her to join in.

This interaction is a good example of the rupture and repair process that has been increasingly recognized as a core change process across a range of therapeutic approaches (Safran, Muran, & Eubanks-Carter, 2011) and through which new ways of managing feelings in relationships can emerge in the context of MBT–C. By looking at what is going on in the moment, the therapist is establishing a sequence and presenting an option of how to deal with the rupture. Furthermore, it invites the child to look at herself from the outside while also trying to stay with the inside experience of the therapist, who is being open and curious. As Tronick (2007) observed, miscommunication and "messiness" are at the heart of the development of the self, and when negative experiences can be repaired in a relationship, it creates increasing levels of self-regulation. The MBT–C therapist can use rupture and repair in the relationship as opportunities to model and engage the child in mentalizing.

Working With Pretend Mode

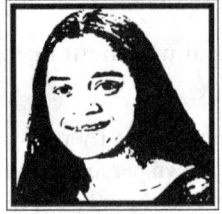

Liza sits down and tells the therapist that her mother has threatened that if she didn't behave better, she couldn't go with the family on a holiday to Spain. Liza says this in a matter-of-fact way, as if she is commenting on the weather. The therapist tries to sympathize with her, saying that that would be an awful situation. Liza laughs out loud and tells the therapist she doesn't mind. She has her own plans. She wants to go on holiday with her friends, taking all her savings and then travel to America to visit Disneyland and go to an Ariana Grande concert. The therapist says, "Wow! You have your own dreams!"

Liza replies that this is not a dream, she really wants to go camping with her friends in America. The therapist senses that Liza is cut off from feeling anything around the rejecting remarks of her mother. She therefore validates Liza's fantasy and tries to exaggerate it even further to try to make her feel something. So again she says, "Wow, you seem to have a lot of plans, Disneyland, Ariana Grande, what else?"

Liza says, "I love America. I really want to go there. I don't like Spain anyway so I wouldn't mind not going with my mother and the others on a holiday."

"Yes," says the therapist, "in fact you might want to just move out of home completely and get your own apartment."

Liza looks a bit shocked and says, "But I'm still only 11—that's not allowed."

Her attention is now firmly on the therapist. "Look," he says, in a much softer voice, "I can hear that it was really horrible when your mum threatened to leave you behind if your behavior doesn't improve. I suppose I'm wondering if it really upset you when she said that?"

Liza suddenly becomes tearful. "She just doesn't see how hard I've been trying," she says, with real feeling. The therapist empathizes with how awful it is when you feel that people don't see all the effort you're putting in to turn things around.

Sometimes as part of a general style of avoiding or cutting off feelings that may be especially hurtful or overwhelming, children can slip into pretend mode. In this state, the child can, for example, pretend not to care about something painful and defensively create grandiose fantasies. The therapist and child are then stuck, unable to address and metabolize the real issue. In the preceding vignette, the therapist finds ways to make contact with Liza and bring her back to the here and now by short-circuiting the pretend mode she has used to avoid her feelings. He does this with a mixture of playful exaggeration and empathy. When children seem disconnected emotionally and operate in pretend mode, the therapist can try to bring them back to the room and help them connect affect and mentalizing in various ways. With Liza, the therapist playfully exaggerates her story to the point where Liza herself is shocked by the therapist, who is doing exactly what she was doing; this allows her the opportunity to see herself from the outside through the therapist. In other words, the therapist is using pretend mode in the service of making Liza aware of how she has used it. This is a high-risk intervention that should be employed with caution and only when there is a good working alliance. It should then be followed by an empathic clarification when the child is back in contact with the therapist.

Pretend mode can also manifest as empty and repetitive play, disconnected from anything meaningful, such as simply lining up toys or painting repetitive patterns or decorative flowers all over the page. This appears to have the function of "papering over" any feelings or thought so as not to feel or think. In these cases, the therapist can try to connect with the child by suggesting that she add specific things to the drawings or the play or by making things happen. For example, the therapist might engage the child in making a messy drawing together, or "messing around," as a way to help the child become unstuck and engaged. The therapist can also try to bring the child back into the room by commenting on her drawing technique or being interested in her way of doing things, imagining what this might be expressing or gradually pulling her actions into imagining with the therapist.

CREATING MENTALIZING NARRATIVES AROUND TRAUMATIC EVENTS

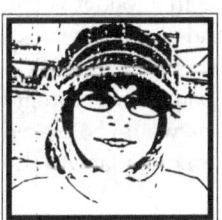 Ruth had been witness to sexual acts in her previous foster family and was not adequately protected by the foster parents. In this particular meeting, the therapist invites Ruth to return to what they talked about in the previous session: witnessing two boys having sex in the foster home. Ruth confirms this, saying with a quiet voice and looking away from the therapist, "Yes they were doing 'it.'"

The therapist responds with the same quiet tone of voice, "In your head you know what you saw, but maybe it is hard to say these things aloud."

Ruth whispers a yes, looking uneasy. The therapist says that maybe it is hard to say things out loud because there were so many thoughts and feelings. Ruth firmly replies with a firm "yes" and puts her hands on her face: "Oh my god."

The therapist repeats, "Oh my god," spontaneously mirroring Ruth's affective state, but with a mix of empathy and concern and also indicating that he is thoughtful and thinking about the experience. Ruth moves uncomfortably in her chair and is quiet. The therapist wonders whether it might be easier if she writes down some feelings and thoughts: "I imagine, Ruth, that you know well what you feel, but it seems to be embarrassing to talk about it with me—did I get it right?"

Ruth nods. He suggests that Ruth draw her feelings. At first Ruth hesitates, then she looks for the right color of paper to start, as if trying to avoid the task. The therapist says it probably won't be a nice drawing, because difficult feelings don't feel nice. Ruth decides she needs a red piece of paper. She draws a face with big eyes and an open mouth, writing in a bubble: "Confused and afraid."

The therapist repeats, "Confused and afraid . . . yes, I can see it in your drawing."

After a short silence, the therapist says, "I am trying to understand this anxious feeling," but then Ruth suddenly writes the word "angry" and explains that is why she chose red. Then she is silent again, and the therapist says calmly, "So some different feelings . . . confused, afraid, and angry."

The therapist again asks permission to talk to Ruth about her feelings, so that he can really understand her. "You write the word 'afraid.' Do you have a sense of what you were afraid of? Sometimes children are afraid of what they have seen. Sometimes they are afraid that it might happen to them." Ruth gets restless on her chair. "I see you are getting restless," the therapist says.

Ruth reads out loud while writing: "I am afraid about what will happen."

"What do you mean?" the therapist asks.

"I am afraid about what will happen," Ruth repeats in a louder voice.

The therapist replies, "Sometimes children are afraid of an angry reaction from the grown-ups who are there to look after them."

Ruth interrupts, saying that her previous foster parents were angry when she told them. She shared that she was afraid she would be placed in yet another foster home, just like 3 years ago. "From one place to the other," says the therapist emphatically.

Ruth adds, "And my brothers, too."

The therapist replies in a compassionate way, saying he knows that Ruth has moved many times and that it has been painful for her. Ruth is letting him know that she is afraid this will happen again. Ruth starts to cry.

In this vignette, Ruth demonstrates that she is capable of staying in touch with the therapist and using his help to express her feelings about what she has seen. She can then articulate her deeper concerns about what this might mean in terms of what is an even deeper trauma for her—that of potentially losing yet another foster family. In putting her feelings into words, she opens the door to being potentially less confused about what happened.

For children like Ruth, part of the value of therapy may be the opportunity to *create a narrative about her life and traumatic experiences* and integrate this into her autobiographical sense of self. Children might have multiple fantasized stories about the conception, birth, trauma, or previous circumstances of their lives, especially when they are an adopted, fostered, or traumatized child. Their ideas, and the ideas of parents, may be both unconscious and conscious, and at times incompatible. At the same time, some children with a difficult start in life or who have experienced trauma find it difficult to integrate these experiences emotionally because they have not had the opportunity and help to put their stories into words. Constructing a coherent narrative about their lives, the trauma and their family or families can help children to explore their experiences in current relationships as well as their narrative about past relationships.

When working with fostered or adopted children, after they have established some capacity for joint attention and affect regulation, the therapist may use questions such as "Do you feel at home?" "What does the word *home* mean to you?" "In what way do you feel that your family belongs together?" "What does the word *family* mean to you?" "How often do you think about your birth parents?" or "What do you call them?" (Muller, Gerits, & Siecker, 2012). The children, too, may have questions about the trauma, such as, "Why did this happen to me?" or "Do my parents still love me?" Exploring such questions can help children to discover a sense of self and other, thereby increasing the capacity to mentalize explicitly and helping them tell a coherent "what makes me, me" story. It is also a way to give meaning to feelings of mourning or sadness, which might be hidden behind an aggressive attitude.

CONCLUSION

In summary, MBT–C involves a process of fluid scaffolding in which the therapist works at a level that is appropriate to the child and seeks to offer the child a new developmental experience in the presence of a therapist who is responsive and guided by curiosity and a genuine attempt to connect. Meeting children where they are—developmentally, cognitively, and emotionally—is central to all the techniques of MBT–C. Especially for children who have had few opportunities to learn about their minds and that of others, a relationship with a therapist who provides a potential space where they can discover who they are and how their minds work may help them open the door to seeing themselves and others in a new way. The journey of psychotherapy, just like the process of development, consists of a fluid and ever-changing road. For the psychotherapist who chooses a relationally based approach such as MBT–C, the most important skill is their own capacity to remain curious and genuine and thus provide the child with an experience in which the expression of feelings, thoughts, and behaviors are freely expressed and looked at from inside and out.

7

WORKING WITH PARENTS FROM A MENTALIZATION-BASED FRAMEWORK

In Chapter 1, we described the qualities and features of a *reflective parenting stance* and how this is evident both in the way that parents are able to imagine the child's perspective and in their ability to interact with the child as a reflective parent. We also described the empirical research that has demonstrated that when parents can take such a reflective stance, it is likely to support their children in terms of emotional growth, security of attachment, and the child's own capacity to thrive. In Chapter 2, we outlined and provided examples of failures and breakdowns in mentalizing in parents, the kind of "vicious cycles of nonmentalizing" that can happen so easily under the pressures of family life and when facing situations or problems that stretch or exceed the abilities even of parents who, in other contexts, have a high capacity to be reflective.

In this chapter, we focus on the work with parents that is offered alongside the child's therapy in time-limited mentalization-based treatment for

http://dx.doi.org/10.1037/0000028-008
Mentalization-Based Treatment for Children: A Time-Limited Approach, by N. Midgley, K. Ensink, K. Lindqvist, N. Malberg, and N. Muller

children (MBT–C). As we described in Chapter 3, regular meetings with the parents or caregivers are always scheduled alongside the direct work with children as part of time-limited MBT–C and, when possible, take place at the same time as the child's meetings but with a separate therapist. In describing our approach, we draw on our own experience and on models of working with parents elaborated by colleagues (e.g., Asen & Fonagy, 2012a, 2012b; Cooper & Redfern, 2016; Etezady & Davis, 2012; Rexwinkel & Verheught-Pleiter, 2008; Suchman, Pajulo, & Mayes, 2013); we have taken particular inspiration from the pioneering work of Slade (2005, 2008).

We consider that in working with parents, reasoned flexibility is important (Slade, 2008). By *reasoned flexibility*, Slade (2008) meant recognizing that when working with parents, it is not always possible to hold to a pure approach, with a fixed, predetermined structure. At times, it may be necessary to see the parents more (or less) often; to offer phone calls or other contact in between meetings, or to set boundaries that limit contact; to see parents only if they come together, or propose that they might work better if they come apart; or to arrange for joint parent–child sessions, or to work only with the parents and not bring the child into the room at all. This variability can make working with parents seem messy, but as long as the therapist holds on to the underlying purpose and aims of the work, Slade reminds us that it remains *reasoned* flexibility, rather than a chaotic response to one crisis after another. (Although, of course, the work can sometimes feel like that too.) Minding parents also means being flexible and responsive to their crises and needs, even when these may be quite different from what the therapist or team might think the focus should be. Especially when working with vulnerable parents who face overwhelming circumstances, such flexibility is essential.

As we hope this chapter will make clear, the work with parents in MBT–C is not done to support the child's therapy alone; it is seen as an integral part of the intervention. Ideally, the sessions should happen regularly enough that they are not simply an occasional opportunity to catch up about the child, but rather provide a space in which some ongoing work and thinking can be done together. The general aim of this aspect of the MBT–C work is to help parents develop a reflective stance, with the following specific goals:

- helping them develop or regain the capacity to look past the child's behavior to his or her experience and mind;
- becoming aware of their own affects and behavior, especially in contexts of conflict when they may lose their mentalizing capacities, which may in turn undermine their child's self-regulation and mentalizing; and
- encouraging parent–child interactions in which the child feels secure and understood and that facilitate motivation, self-regulation, basic self-knowledge, and mentalizing.

Airplane safety instructions remind parents that in the case of an emergency, they should put on their own oxygen mask first before helping their children with theirs; likewise, when a child is referred for therapeutic help, it is essential that we do not neglect the parents' needs. This is not only because the parents play an important role in helping their child but also because any changes that children make in therapy will be maintained only if the environment in which they spend the majority of their day helps sustain the changes. In their reframing of therapeutic change in terms of restoring epistemic trust, Fonagy and Allison (2014) made the important point that the emergence of robust mentalizing in therapy is only the start of the process of change. In the context of adult therapy, they wrote,

> In the past modifications of the patient's social world were felt to fall outside the concerns of therapy. It is possible, however, that effective treatments depend as much on ensuring that the patient's social environment is benign as on ensuring a similar emotional tone in the consulting room. (p. 378)

If this is true of work with adults, it is even more so when working with children. Helping parents improve mentalizing capacities under relational stress supports the development of mentalizing capacities in children. In this chapter, we hope to illustrate ways in which MBT–C therapists can promote parents' capacity to do all of these things and thereby to support children's renewed capacity to learn from the significant adults in their lives.

Our basic assumption at the outset is that most parents have a deep wish to do right by their children, to be the best parents they can be, regardless of their own difficulties, whether these be financial stress, psychological difficulties, or their own childhood histories of relational trauma or neglect. However, many parents struggle despite their best intentions not to fall back and repeat patterns from the past, and they often need help to become the parents they wish to be and develop skills in thinking and relating to their children in ways that can help their children develop and flourish. Parenting is arguably one of the most important and challenging human endeavors, and also one of the most rewarding and meaningful; but parents of children who have been referred to clinical services frequently require help to develop ways of relating to their children and supporting their development. This can be especially true when parents did not experience such relationships as children and thus have few, if any, internal role models to guide them.

To add to the challenge, it may be more difficult for parents of children with emotional or behavioral difficulties to mentalize about their child because such difficulties can evoke uncomfortable and sometimes overwhelming affects, such as anger or helplessness, that interfere with the parent's capacity to mentalize. A child's temperament may be very different from that of the parent or his siblings, making it hard for the parent to identify and understand how the child experiences the world. Sometimes this contributes to a perception that the child is purposely behaving badly, simply to be naughty or provoke the people around them.

Troubled and externalizing children can strain even the most thoughtful and loving parents and erode couple relationships, especially when one parent shoulders a larger burden of care or when parents disagree about how to respond to the child's difficulties. Negative feelings toward one's own child can be seen as taboo—difficult to admit even to oneself. Guilt about such "forbidden feelings" can lead to denial, hindering mentalization and constructive problem-solving. Therefore, an important aim of the work with parents is to help them mentalize about their own feelings to better understand their reactions to their child and to become more flexible and open.

THE MENTALIZING STANCE IN WORK WITH PARENTS

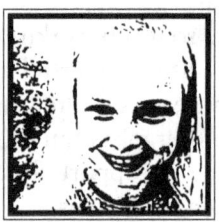

Belinda's mother, Mrs. C, comes to an individual session with the therapist to discuss difficulties she is experiencing in her relationship with her daughter. She tells the therapist that she just needs ways of talking to Belinda that are effective and confides that she frequently fears she is going to "lose her mind" with Belinda, especially when she can't get her out of the house in the morning. The therapist empathizes with how awful it must feel when Mrs. C feels she's losing her mind. Mrs. C agrees but then insists that what she needs urgently is not sympathy but strategies to work with Belinda. The therapist accepts this, apologizes, and agrees that it is important for Mrs. C to leave the session feeling she has some better ideas to handle the morning situation. He asks whether Mrs. C would find it helpful to tell him about one of the times recently when things have been hard, and then they could think about it together and see if they can come up with some ideas for what would help next time. Mrs. C says yes, that would be helpful, and starts telling the therapist about a difficult incident from that morning.

As the therapist listens, he sometimes slows things down, asking Mrs. C to talk him through it one step at a time, and checks out what was going on for Mrs. C at a given moment. Sometimes he interjects with supportive comments, such as, "Yes, that does sound tough!" or "Yes, parents often say they struggle when their children do that." As they continue and begin to make sense of what happened that day, Mrs. C seems calmer and more relaxed, and her voice becomes less insistent and panicky. The therapist also begins to express some curiosity about what Mrs. C thinks was going on with her daughter at the time: "So when you said that, how did she respond?" or "What do you think she felt when you said that?" Mrs. C gradually starts to become a little more reflective, and she and the therapist continue to think together about that morning's events.

In Chapter 4, we spoke about the importance of the therapist's *mentalizing stance*, including the basic therapeutic presence of the therapist (i.e., a basic helping orientation; authenticity; being nonjudgmental, genuine, and accepting); an interest in the mind, not just behavior; curiosity and the not-knowing (or inquisitive) stance; and the importance of monitoring misunderstandings. All these are equally relevant to our work with parents as they are to our work with children in therapy, but some aspects of the mentalizing stance are especially important or may take on particular significance in this part of the work.

First of all, it must be acknowledged that many parents do not bring their child to therapy because they want the child to "become more reflective." This is not necessarily the highest thing on parents' agenda when they are struggling with looking after a child who may be having tantrums, not sleeping at night, can't get on with peers, is constantly in tears, or who struggles every morning to get out of bed and get on the bus to school. In most cases—and quite rightly so—parents are likely to be seeking professional help because they want help changing their child's behavior or reducing distress, or, at the very least, they are seeking solid, professional advice on how they can better manage the situation. When Mrs. C starts the session just described by talking about the difficulties she is having getting her daughter to school in the morning, she appears to find it irritating when the therapist simply empathizes with her feelings. The therapist quickly appreciates that he needs to take this concern seriously and apologizes for getting it wrong. (This is not to say that being empathic is wrong but that at that moment, he hadn't offered what Mrs. C needed.) The therapist needs to help Mrs. C feel that her worries are being heard and that coming to therapy can make a difference in the problems at home. In suggesting that they focus on a particular incident, the therapist is trying in the first instance to help regulate Mrs. C's affect and to *come alongside her*, using the word *we* to make clear that the two of them will collaborate together to come up with solutions. Once Mrs. C feels her concerns are being taken seriously, she is able to calm down, and at that stage, a more reflective atmosphere is created.

Slade (2008) suggests that the first aim of work with parents from a mentalizing perspective is the creation of a *play space*, an environment where the parent can "feel safe enough to mentalize, to envision, name, and play with mental states" (p. 221). Doing so relies on our communicating to parents the importance that they have in supporting their child and our respect for their experiences as a parent. Paradoxically, it may sometimes require us to start by focusing on behavior, if that is what the parent is struggling with, as a basis for creating a context in which the parent feels heard and safe enough to become curious about mental states. Therapists can model the process of stopping, thinking, and wondering for parents with our mentalizing stance during sessions. Parents need to feel understood and taken seriously in their concerns and their struggles. As Pally and Popek (2012) put it, the therapist needs to hold a delicate balance: "*emphasizing* a parent's strengths and *empathizing* with weaknesses" (p. 53, italics in original). With regard to the latter, this may mean that there are times when we do not confront what we may consider "bad" parenting practices, even when we may have concerns about how they are affecting the child. For example, when a parent tells us that her daughter "gave me a look I knew was disrespectful, so I grounded her for a week," we may have our own ideas about whether the mother has interpreted her child's behavior correctly and might have our own views on whether the punishment she imposed was appropriate. However, our initial response may need to empathize with how awful it is as a parent when you feel that your child doesn't show respect. Such a response helps to validate the parent's experience and will hopefully make her feel heard, recognized, and supported. It may only be sometime later that we can then come back to the incident itself and work together to think about other possible meanings of the child's "disrespectful" look and explore alternative ways the parent could have responded.

This example speaks to the issue of how a therapist working with parents in MBT–C can hold a not-knowing position, especially in the face of requests for advice or when hearing about parenting behaviors that do not seem productive. In such situations, we as therapists may feel a strong pull to make suggestions or to come up with an "expert" view on what a child needs to support his development. As described in Chapter 4, the not-knowing stance is not the same as knowing nothing: As therapists, we have expertise and ideas, and sharing our knowledge and making suggestions is a perfectly valid aspect of working with parents in MBT–C. But it is only done at the point when the parents' mentalizing is online so that these ideas can be accepted as another perspective, one that can be thought about, explored, and either accepted or rejected. If expert advice is offered when the parents' mentalizing is offline, and they are perhaps demanding that you come up with an immediate solution (teleological mode) or telling you that they know exactly why their child behaved in a certain way (psychic equivalence), then the advice is unlikely to be of much help. As Rexwinkel and Verheugt-Pleiter (2008) recognized, when parents are operating in a nonmentalizing mode, "they often follow child-rearing advice much too literally because, although their need for advice is great, the framework for applying it as it was meant to be applied is not there" (p. 74). The parent therapist in MBT–C is therefore encouraged to resist the temptation to jump in and problem-solve, while validating the parents' wish to find an answer about what they should do (Pally & Popek, 2012).

Many parents come to therapy with a fear that a therapist is going to point out their failures as a parent (Slade, 2008), something they may already feel guilty about. We need to work to avoid confirming these preconceptions if we are going to help foster a reflective stance in which parents can experience the way that developing curiosity about their child's mind and behaviors will help them build a stronger relationship with their child and find creative solutions to the practical challenges of being a parent.

There is also a risk that, with MBT–C, it may sound as if we are only interested in thoughts and feelings and that behavior doesn't matter. This is not what we mean when we describe the importance of maintaining a mentalizing stance. At the end of the day, the work with parents is not going to be successful if the parents do not come away from it feeling that it has helped them with the difficulties that first spurred them to seek help. To make sure this is kept in mind, we have found it can be helpful to use an idea suggested by Haugvik (2013), who, at the end of each session, asks parents two questions: "What do you feel has been most important for you in our talk today?" and "What do you feel has been most important in relation to the child in this session?" (p. 507). Haugvik points out that, in addition to providing an opportunity to check that the work being done with the parents is relevant and meaningful to them, these questions are also a way of stimulating mentalizing capacity in the parents by encouraging them to think about what has gone on in that day's session—from their own perspective and that of their child. And of course, if the answer to these questions is "nothing," then this is extremely important feedback for the therapist, who will need to acknowledge this failure and invite the parents to work together next time to ensure that the same thing doesn't happen again.

WORKING WITH STRENGTHS, ENCOURAGING OBSERVATION, AND PROMOTING PLAY

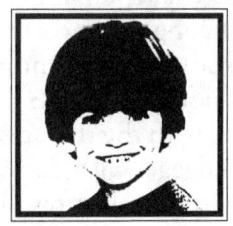

Mohammed's father, Mr. D, comes to the second parent meeting with his new partner, Ms. L. Since Mohammed's accident, she has been his primary caregiver when he is staying with them, with Mr. D getting involved mostly as a disciplinarian. For this reason, the therapist suggested at the previous meeting that Mr. D try to find half an hour during the week to sit down with Mohammed and play with him. She suggested that Mr. D simply follow the play and not try to steer it or make the game "educational." She asked him to observe as closely as possible and come back this week and tell her how it went and what he noticed.

Ms. L begins by teasingly saying that it took several reminders on her part for Mr. D to find the time to do this, but in the end, Mr. D sat down with Mohammed over the weekend, and they had played with some LEGO blocks together. "In my family, my father would never have sat down and played with me!" laughs Mr. D, and when the therapist asks what it was like for him to do this, he says that it felt odd at first, but in the end he enjoyed it. He explains how they built two spaceships and then had some races around the room. "I didn't know how much Mohammed knows about science and space travel—he's a real expert." He goes on to say that the play got a little bit overheated, especially when the spaceships crashed into the furniture, but he remembered what the therapist had said last week and tried not to tell Mohammed to stop.

"How do you think that was for Mohammed?" asks the therapist, and Mr. D says that he seemed to have enjoyed it—"He's probably used to me telling him off recently, so I guess it was nice for him that I wasn't just doing that . . . and nice for me too, to be honest."

The therapist compliments Mr. D on his sensitivity to what this had been like for Mohammed and asks whether Ms. L had noticed a difference that day. Ms. L says that after the game, they'd actually had a peaceful evening. Asked if she had any thoughts about why that might be, Ms. L says, "Well, it just changed the atmosphere in the house a bit—and I guess playing at spaceship crashes isn't a thousand miles from car crashes, so maybe it was good for Mohammed to play out some of his worries."

Mr. D looks surprised and says he hadn't thought of it that way at all. He asks the therapist, with genuine curiosity, if she thinks Mohammed's play was connected to the car accident.

The work with parents in the MBT–C model is, as much as possible, a strengths-based approach, starting with *confirming and validating* what parents are doing well. Reinforcing parents' attempts to understand their child during the session helps them to feel at ease and understood, in turn fostering an atmosphere of mutual collaboration and exploration. This can make it possible for parents to develop increased curiosity about their children's inner worlds. For example, when working with a young single mother who spends hours helping her son with homework after a long day's work, even though this often leads to arguments, it can help to start by commenting on the conscientiousness and effort this takes on the mother's part. Starting in this way may help her be more receptive to thinking with the therapist but also affirms her strengths, helps her feel capable, and engages with the side of her that is resourceful. The mother may then work with the therapist, helping her discover and develop her other capacities as a mother, for example, to become more thoughtful about her son and to explore what is leading the two of them to end up arguing so often.

The parent therapist takes an active stance to support the parent and works alongside, or "behind," the parent, trying to see things from his or her perspective (Lieberman, Padrón, Van Horn, & Harris, 2005). The therapist takes an active role and does not hesitate to share information when this can be helpful to the parent. The therapist is mindful of what the parent will be receptive to and be able to use and takes care to work in the parent's *zone of proximal development* (Vygotsky, 1978). By this, we mean trying to offer only what the parent is able to make use of at that moment or intervening only one step ahead of where she is currently operating, helping her to achieve what is within her reach. The therapist takes care to build on the strengths of the parent and make sure that she feels her efforts and struggles are acknowledged. The therapist also highlights successful mentalizing, ensuring that parents see how doing this well makes a difference to their relationship with their child.

In the vignette with Mr. D, the therapist actively "marks" the moment when Mr. D shows curiosity about his child's experience and reflects on what it may have felt like for him to be engaging with Mohammed in a way that was more playful. The therapist had suggested that they find time to play together because she hoped this would create a different kind of interaction between father and son, during a period when Mr. D had been spending a lot of time taking on the role of disciplining Mohammed for his aggressive outbursts. As described in earlier chapters, this joint play would also provide Mohammed with opportunities to develop his own mentalizing capacities, build relationships, and, as Ms. L perceptively realized, also to revisit in a safe context experiences that had been upsetting and distressing. By the end of this brief review of the play activity, Mr. D was demonstrating a genuine curiosity about his son's mind, in a way that boded well for the ongoing work in therapy.

By suggesting to Mr. D that he should not direct the play with Mohammed but simply try to follow his son's lead, the therapist was also trying to invite this boy's father to develop his own curiosity about his son's experiences. In so doing, Mr. D was able to see an aspect of his son that he did not usually notice and also found time to reflect on what it was like for him as a father to have this different kind of interaction—one that hadn't been part of his own experience of being parented as a child. One effective way in which MBT–C therapists can help this process of self-observation in the parent is by helping the parent take a developmental perspective— that is, encouraging and reinforcing attempts in parents that indicate a curiosity and awareness of the role of maturation and experience in learning to think, perceive, and feel about relationships in more complex ways.

Cooper and Redfern (2016), in their book for parents on reflective parenting, described what they call the *Parent App*, which they suggested can be helpful for parents who want to attune to their child's experience and improve their relationship. This Parent App is not something to download onto your phone (or at least it isn't yet!) but rather a stance that parents are encouraged to take, made up of three components:

- *Attention*—To become curious about a child's behavior, a parent first needs to pay attention, stepping back to watch, listen, and be curious about the child.
- *Perspective-taking*—Instead of assuming that the child sees the world in the same way as his parents, the parents try to step back and imagine how the child may be seeing things. As Cooper and Redfern (2016) put it, "Your child may be behaving in a way that is unreasonable, but for a reason that is entirely reasonable" (p. 76).
- *Providing empathy*—This involves imaginatively standing alongside the child, showing that you are able to connect with their experience of an event.

In the preceding vignette, Mr. D's therapist is in essence trying to work with him to promote this stance. Finding creative ways to help parents become attentive to their child in itself stimulates curiosity. As Cooper and Redfern (2016) put it, "The impact of being attentive to what your baby or child is doing, thinking and feeling cannot be overestimated" (p. 71) because learning to observe and become curious about a child's behavior is the first step toward being able to understand it better. Once parents are curious about their child, they are likely to become less critical and less absolute in their understanding of what may be going on. At this stage, the therapist can actively encourage parents to explore situations from different perspectives. This does not only have to include the child's perspective. For example, some parents find it a very powerful experience to be asked, "If your best friend/your own parent were here now, what do you think she would say about what is going on?" Asking parents to step out of their own shoes and look at a situation from another perspective often has therapeutic value in and of itself. It can then be much easier for parents to be empathic with their child even if they may not like or agree with what the child is doing.

One way of inviting a different perspective is to *explore the parent's own experiences of being a child*, as Mr. D did spontaneously when he commented on how his father would never have played with him in this way. There is some debate in the literature about how appropriate or necessary it is, when working with parents, to actively explore the parents' own experiences of being parented as part of the process of increasing self-awareness and self-observation (Whitefield & Midgley, 2015). In time-limited MBT–C, there is no requirement or expectation that parents be asked to speak about their own childhood experiences, but there are times when a parent may spontaneously refer back to his own experience of being parented or the therapist may choose to ask about such experiences. This may be the first time parents have the opportunity to think about themselves as parents and what role models they had in this capacity. It may help them to articulate what they struggle with and what kind of parent they want to be, as well as to think about this from an intergenerational perspective and in terms of the stories of their lives (Siegel & Hartzell, 2014). Sometimes it may help parents with difficult attachment histories and trauma to have a therapist who is perceptive and compassionate regarding their struggles to be resilient as parents, to address both the "ghosts in the nursery" that may cast doubts about their parenting (Fraiberg, Adelson, & Shapiro, 1975) and the "angels" that are there to help them (Lieberman et al., 2005). It can also provide opportunities to think about ways in which their own child may be different from what they were like as children, especially if there is a strong overidentification with the child's experiences. In having such discussions, however, the focus remains on helping to support parental reflective functioning in the here and now.

IDENTIFYING TRIGGERS FOR STRONG EMOTIONS

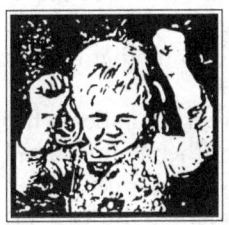

The previous week, Anne's mother, Mrs. H, had been describing how difficult dinnertime was at home and had said to the parent therapist, "If you could see it, you'd understand what I mean." The therapist had been curious about what Mrs. H thought he might see that he didn't get from Mrs. H describing the situation to him, but after exploring this further, he had suggested that if it would be helpful, Mrs. H would be welcome to video one of the meals at home and bring it to review together at their next meeting. Mrs. H had said that she'd find this really helpful.

The following week, Anne's mother brings a recording of the two of them eating together, and the therapist suggests she pick a short extract to show him, which sums up what she wants the therapist to know about the difficulties they have. He asks if it is OK if either of them can pause the video at any time when they think something important happened, and Mrs. H agrees to this. The two of them sit together and watch, and at certain moments either Mrs. H or the therapist presses Pause. At first Anne's mother does this to make comments such as, "Look, that's what she's always doing!" or "Can you see how rude she's being?" The therapist responds by empathizing with the difficultly of the situation, adding that if he were the parent at that moment, he might also really struggle to keep his cool.

At one point, the therapist observes a shift in Mrs. H's affect, so he pauses and wonders about it. Mrs. H speaks of noticing that Anne was trying to get her attention the whole time, and that this "always winds me up." The two of them go back and replay that sequence, and the therapist notices that at first Anne seems to have found something she's interested in that she wants to show Mrs. H. When she doesn't get her mother's attention right away, her voice becomes whinier, and then Mrs. H gets annoyed. "Yes, that's what happens all the time!" exclaims Mrs. H.

The therapist helps Mrs. H explore her own reaction to this, and then asks her what face she thinks Anne sees when her mother gets wound up like this? Mrs. H says that she's not sure—probably a pretty exhausted one. The therapist says, "I imagine this was at the end of your working day, and I can understand that you were probably very tired."

Mrs. H goes back to the video and plays it back once again. "You know I didn't really have the energy to speak to Anne right then, but she probably just wanted to show me something." The therapist stays with this and a little later asks Mrs. H what face she'd want Anne to see when she looks up at her. Mrs. H isn't sure and says when she's that tired, she can't find the right words to say anything. She asks the therapist if he can suggest something. The therapist says that some parents he has spoken to, when they are just too exhausted to speak, have tried to make contact with their children by just touching them. He explains that touching is sometimes more important than words. Mrs. H agrees to give this a try, adding that this is very different from the way her own mother used to handle things.

At the next session, Anne's mother comes in with a big smile on her face. She tells the therapist that a miracle happened: When Anne started demanding her attention, Mrs. H made contact with her by touching her arm. She then told Anne that she'd give her attention when the food was ready and they were sitting down at the table. Anne stopped whining, and had even waited a minute before trying to get her attention again. In response, Mrs. H could caress her hair, and thank her for being patient, and they both felt connected.

Identifying the usual "bumpy roads" (Malberg, 2015) or "hot spots" (Slade, 2008) that are the common battlegrounds where children and parents seem to have the most difficulty in their interactions is of great value in work with parents. Although parents may sometimes want to speak in generalities ("my child always does X" or "what usually happens is Y"), getting down to the nitty-gritty and exploring a particular incident where things have been difficult can pave the way and help the therapist and parents develop an understanding of how and when mentalizing breaks down. These incidents often turn out to be examples of the vicious cycles of nonmentalizing that we described in Chapter 2, where parents and child enter patterns of relating in which nonmentalizing in one arouses nonmentalizing in the other.

Examining a specific example is usually more therapeutically productive than speaking about how this happens in general or "all the time."

Often, the first step in reviewing these "hot-spot" moments involves a *process of sequencing or microanalysis* in which the parent and therapist jointly reconstruct what happened. Prompted by the therapist's interest and request for clarification (e.g., "And then what happened?", "Let me see whether I have this right."), the therapist and parent clarify and elaborate the emotional and behavioral sequence in the interactions until they have a clear picture and frame-by-frame, slow-motion movie of exactly what triggers and escalates interpersonal breakdowns. Slowing down interactions that are often so affectively charged that they are remembered as a blur helps parents mentally observe their own behavior from the outside and think about their child's reactions, thus paving the way to understand breakdowns and behaviors that "happen for no reason." This can be a springboard for the therapist to invite curiosity about what was going on for all of the people involved in the interaction.

By inviting parents to "stop and rewind" in this way (a technique we described in Chapter 6), the therapist helps them understand the sequence underlying repeated or common cycles of nonmentalizing in their family. This is the first step in helping them regulate and adjust their own behavior, and then being able to catch themselves when they react in a way that will escalate the child's dysregulation, rather than help them to regulate. The therapist can also bring in her own thoughts and perspectives on what may have been going on, checking with the parents and asking them to consider these different perspectives from an inquisitive and curious position. In this way, the therapist also models the path to mentalizing and thinking together about why each person reacts a certain way and noticing where mentalizing breaks down.

Verbal accounts of incidents from outside the session can be used with the stop-and-rewind technique, but in some cases, it can be powerful to work with video material. Video is now widely used in many intervention approaches, especially in parent–infant psychotherapy and attachment-based interventions with high-risk parent–child dyads, but it may not be the right strategy for all parents. When parents are fragile and have a great deal of guilt and paranoia regarding inadequate parenting, some work on building their sense of competence or helping them with immediate difficulties may be a priority; video may be too exposing and threatening. Likewise, there is a risk that parents may want to use video as a way of showing up or humiliating their child (e.g., by showing the therapist how awful their child's behavior really is). When used in this way, it is unlikely to be helpful.

Video can serve as a way of explicitly helping parents increase self–other observational skills and recognize examples of positive mentalizing. This can lead to an increase in reflective functioning in the parent as well as to a feeling of mutual collaboration between the therapist and the parent. Difficult interactions, in which mentalizing may have broken down, can also be a focus for review. Video can be invaluable in providing an opportunity for parents to look at themselves from a distance in a way that is much more challenging, if not impossible, when in the midst of a situation, especially if it is an affectively charged one.

The therapist can ask questions while watching the video, for example: "What do you think your child was trying to say with that behavior right there?" "What were you feeling when your child was behaving like that?" In this way, the therapist can shift between inviting mentalizing of self and the other. These questions help in the process of making links between what can and can't be seen and to concretely illustrate the concept of the opacity of minds.

In MBT–C, we use video feedback with parents to

- highlight examples of positive mentalizing, helping parents to see what they are doing well and how that can support the relationship they have with their child;
- provide an opportunity to look at "hot-spot" interactions from a distance and when not emotionally activated, using the more reflective and observing stance naturally activated by the video to increase awareness of self and other;
- increase awareness of affects and their impact, especially the parents' own negative affects and intensity of anger that they maybe not have been aware of;
- increase curiosity about the child's experience underlying their behavior, thus preparing the ground for adapting their reactions so they can help the child regulate; and
- observe and understand the sequence of interactions that increase child dysregulation.

With some parents, the use of video may not be possible or welcome; in these cases, a *journal or self-monitoring log* can be useful to facilitate the development of self-awareness and self-regulation (monitoring and reflecting). Especially in working with parents whose capacity to mentalize is easily lost, it can be helpful to keep a log that activates a self-monitoring function and engages the more cognitive, reflective part of the parent. It is useful to encourage parents to use the journal right after a difficult moment or conflict with their child, while acknowledging the influence of strong affect on their perceptions of the child and themselves at that moment. It requires a good therapeutic alliance and basic trust for parents to share what they may feel are embarrassing or forbidden thoughts and feelings about themselves as parents and their children that come up during painful and helpless exchanges. However, looking at these entries together during a meeting can help facilitate the task of self-observation in a safe and contained environment and encourage parents' development of self-monitoring.

WORKING WITH PARENTS IN CONFLICT

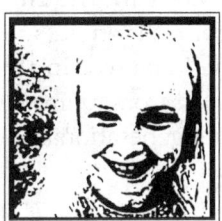 Belinda's main caregivers, Mrs. C and Grandma, are discussing her rude vocabulary. Grandma says that it isn't surprising given that Mrs. C is not careful with the TV programs she allows Belinda to watch. This sets off Mrs. C, and she shouts at her mother that she is old-fashioned and controlling. Grandma shouts back, accusing her daughter of undermining her just to punish her. The therapist puts up his hands to indicate that they should stop, and when this is ignored, he stands up and uses his hands to indicate that they should "simmer down." With a firm voice, he interrupts the two of them and says, "I'm going to stop you there, because I don't think it helps anyone if I let the two of you shout at each other."

They stop shouting, but the tension remains high. "If you think that was shouting," says Grandma, "you should hear her at home when she really shouts—Belinda goes and locks herself in the bathroom."

"Well that's helpful to know," says the therapist, "and maybe we'll need to come back later and think about what it might be like for Belinda when the two of you are arguing. Because for me, that did feel like shouting, and when it is like that, I find it really difficult to think. And if I can't think properly, I'm probably not going to be able to help much."

Mrs. C and Grandma look at each other, and the tension in the room decreases slightly. "So are you two both OK," the therapist goes on, "if I step in and stop you like that when the volume goes up?"

Mrs. C and Grandma both nod. "Thank you," says the therapist, "and thanks also for explaining to me that compared with what goes on at home, you don't consider that shouting. . . . Is that how you see it too, Mrs. C?"

Mrs. C nods again, and says yes, at home they sometimes shout so loud, the neighbors knock on the door and check to see if everything is OK. "Well, that's really important for me to know," says the therapist, "and is that how the two of you want it to be?"

Mrs. C and Grandma both shake their heads. "And is it how you want it to be for Belinda?"

Again, they both shake their heads, but this time Mrs. C also looks tearful.

Conflict is inherent in humans and thus in families, but divorce and the dissolution of the original family unit often trigger deep and profound anxiety and anger around loss of and access to children, abandonment, future financial security, and division of family resources. This frequently activates nonmentalizing, coercive patterns in the separating parents (Nyberg & Hertzmann, 2014). However, it is not only in the context of divorce that therapists encounter conflict. As illustrated by the preceding vignette, conflicts around parenting often become a way in which parents and family members caring for the child can express their fears and other painful affects. When a parent is afraid, angry, or confused, her mentalizing capacity is likely to become impaired. In this section, we think about how to work with parents in conflict from a time-limited MBT–C perspective in parent sessions. This includes intergenerational conflict, as in our example, or conflict within a parental couple.

One of the main questions that emerges in the context of family conflict is how ready are the parents or caregivers to engage collectively in the process of making meaning of the child's behavior and their own. This will affect the therapeutic framework chosen for each case—namely, would the therapist favor parallel sessions at first to explore the individual sources of conflict and the impact on the child, or would she meet with both parents and other significant caregivers all at once? For example, with separated or divorced parents where there is a history of coercive mentalizing patterns, it may not be suitable to meet with both at the same time because their own relational agenda may take over. That said, witnessing and assessing such interactions is always important in the context of the initial assessment. Sometimes it can be important for separated or divorced parents to come together and create a shared perspective of their child. The main aim always remains to find the best setting in which parents can learn to mentalize each other and the child in a way that will contribute to a more coherent and predictable relational experience for the child, one in which they can feel seen and heard.

The first step is generally to provide parents with such an experience in the context of parent sessions. For instance, during sessions with parents, feelings can become overheated, and it can be challenging to remain calm when angry parents are shouting at each other and assuming threatening postures. Trying to enter into a discussion about the meaning of what is being said (e.g., Grandma's comment that Mrs. C is doing this "to hurt her") is almost certain to have little value. When the level of conflict and arousal is high in the room, our own capacity for mentalizing is likely to be inhibited, so it is important to try to stop the interaction before the therapist becomes overwhelmed, sometimes using what MBT workers with families have called, somewhat jokingly, the "mentalizing hand" (Asen & Fonagy, 2012a). In doing so, it can be helpful to use your own experience as the therapist in the room to explain why you are trying to stop the parents and get them to "simmer down"; this can introduce the idea that behaviors have an impact on others and that others may experience our behavior very differently to how we see it ourselves.

By inviting parents to simmer down and introducing our capacity to be reflective about what is going on in the room, we try to model *thinking while feeling*. In retrospect, when reviewing interactions like this, the therapist can sometimes introduce an element of psychoeducation about what happens when we get into dysregulated states or use such reviewing to help the parents recognize patterns and check whether they are ones that the parents want to repeat. Parents themselves usually do not want these interactions to continue, so this can be the basis for deepening the therapeutic alliance, with a shared goal about areas that parents would like to work on.

Whenever the emotional temperature in a session becomes high, as in the preceding example, it is important to acknowledge it and, once things have simmered down, invite participants to think about what happened. The stop-and-rewind method helps to cool off the interaction so that those involved can reflect on the sequence of thoughts and feelings that emerged before and during the moment when things became heated, allowing the situation to be mentalized. In the preceding vignette, Grandma raised the issue of how Belinda reacts to the shouting in the house; as this demonstrates, it is often easy for a child to get lost in parents' minds when they are in the midst of an argument. Thus, having a space and an opportunity to consider what Belinda's experience might be when her mother and grandma are arguing, as well as to slow down, pause, and wonder about what is going on between them, can be extremely helpful. However, when it is clear that parental or caregiver conflict is chronic and ongoing, it is likely that time-limited work as part of MBT–C may not be sufficient, and a referral to some form of couple therapy may be required (Hertzmann & Abse, 2010). This can sometimes take place alongside the time-limited MBT–C, so that the child's therapy is not interrupted and the MBT–C parent meetings can focus on their role as parents in responding to their child's needs.

WORKING WITH FOSTER PARENTS

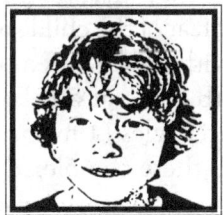 John's foster parents are speaking to the therapist about their concerns about what will happen in terms of John's permanent placement with them. His biological father has petitioned the court for visitation, and John's behavior, the foster parents say, has deteriorated since then. "It is like they don't want this boy to have peace of mind. . . . Don't they understand, they are going to drive him crazy?" The therapist asks

them whether they have spoken with John about this at all. "I tried," says Mr. F, "but he told me to piss off and mind my own business—in fact, he told me that if we stopped him from seeing his mom, he'd never speak to me again."

They explain that John's social worker also spoke to them, and when they voiced their concerns, they felt that the social worker was quite critical of them and implied that they didn't know what was best for John. "I felt like telling her to come and live with John for a week," says Mrs. F, "and then tell us who knows best."

Although the approach to working with foster parents in time-limited MBT–C is similar to that with other parents, there are a number of specific issues that this work can raise. First of all, as described in Chapter 2, many of the children who come into the care system have not had the experience, in their early years, of a parent who is able to notice or think about what is going on in their minds or to offer marked or contingent mirroring. As children, they may have had many experiences in which their intentions were misread, there were negative attributions about their behavior, or there was extreme inconsistency in how their attachment needs were met. In turn, these children may be avoidant of their dependency needs; they may appear highly controlling and domineering in ways that invite rejection from adults and may even be frightening. Or they may be prone to hyperarousal, behave in a way that can be seen as "attention-seeking," or be indiscriminate in their attachments (Taylor, 2012). These children, like John and Ruth in this book, are likely to have negative views of themselves, often believing that they are unlovable, shameful, and worthy of rejection.

Research has suggested that some foster parents may have variable levels of reflective functioning, with limitations specifically in aspects that may be most important for effective fostering (Bunday, Dallos, Morgan, & McKenzie, 2015). It is not surprising, then, that fostered children and their carers often struggle to understand each other; furthermore, foster parents may well have trouble dealing with the highly rejecting behavior that these children may display or struggle with their incapacity to show emotional responsiveness (Muller, Gerits, & Siecker, 2012). Some carers may struggle to set limits out of a wish to make up for the lack of love and care that they imagine the child experienced when they were younger or possibly out of fear of the child's aggression and anger. In other instances, the carers might withdraw from emotional engagement with the child in their care, dealing with them at a behavioral level, often ending up in power struggles, leading to cycles of misbehavior and punishment (Jacobsen, Ha, & Sharp, 2015). All these complex dynamics can easily get played out in the systems around the child as well, as seems to be the case with John in the preceding vignette, where there is mutual blame and anger among the child, foster parents, and social work team. In these situations, foster parents often have to endure the lack of permanency and the unexpected demands of a system that, although designed to support them, often turns to measures that result in an exacerbation of nonmentalizing responses to the needs of both carers and children. As a result, foster parents may end up feeling frustrated, angry, puzzled, or deeply distressed.

In considering how best to support foster parents in the context of a mentalizing approach, Cooper and Redfern (2016) talked about the need to have an "enhanced Parent App" (p. 126). By this, they meant a stance toward parenting with an increased focus on perspective-taking, given how hard it can be for foster parents if a child sees them, as John does (at least momentarily), as uncaring or nasty or treats them with distrust and hostility. The parent therapist may therefore need to work especially hard at helping the foster parents see things from the child's perspective, and in many cases this can be helped (if foster parents do not already have this knowledge) with a degree of psychoeducation about attachment and trauma and the impact of early maltreatment and abuse on how children see the world and relate to it.

Managing problematic behaviors is one area with which foster parents often struggle, given the extreme emotion dysregulation they are frequently challenged to respond to. They can sometimes feel caught between advice to take an entirely behavioral approach (e.g., time outs, reward systems) or having to simply empathize and see things from the child's perspective, which can sometimes leave the foster parents feeling that they are giving the child carte blanche to behave as they like. Drawing on the work of Golding and Hughes (e.g., Golding, 2015; Hughes, 2000), Cooper and Redfern (2016) suggested that the concept of "Two Hands" is compatible with a mentalizing approach. The Two Hands approach involves managing behavior on the one hand, while seeking to understand it on the other. For example, when John was rude to his foster father and told him to "piss off," it would be possible to encourage Mr. F to consider both *whether* and *how* to respond when spoken to in this way, while remaining curious about *why* John may have spoken in that way. As Cooper and Redfern put it, "it is easier to influence others when they have a feeling of being understood and connected with [and] nowhere is this more important than when disciplining your child" (p. 107).

In addition to the meetings that are offered to foster parents, the parent therapist may also need to liaise with teachers, social workers, and other allied professionals. The aim of this work is to help "mentalize the system" (Bevington, Fuggle, & Fonagy, 2015) by offering a new version of the child's and, in this case, the parents' behavior, one that introduces an inquisitive style alongside a developmental and trauma-informed perspective. As with individuals, when the members of the profession network around a child in care are under pressure, they may lose the capacity to remain reflective. If the network cannot sustain such pressure, they are likely to act out in unthinking ways, often making rash decisions that may not be based on holding in mind the child's perspective (Emanuel, 2002; Taylor, 2012). When operating in a nonmentalizing, teleological mode of this sort, there can be a powerful pressure to "do something." Although action may well be necessary, the therapist may need to make use of mentalizing techniques such as slowing down, stop and review, or simmering down with members of the network around the child to help restart more mentalizing interactions and ensure that any action taken is thoughtful and based on the capacity to take the foster child's perspective (Wood, Brasnett, Lassri, Fearon, & Midgley, 2015).

COMING TO THE END OF THE WORK WITH PARENTS

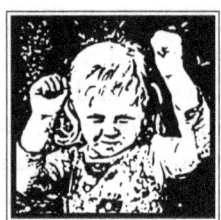

By the time the meetings with Mrs. H come to an end, there are marked improvements in her personal and professional life, and she appears to feel much more confident about her ability to control herself and see herself as a competent parent who is able to understand, if not change, her daughter, Anne. However, in the review meeting, Mrs. H becomes distressed when the therapist reflects on her progress and wonders whether it is time to think of moving toward ending treatment. Mrs. H says that she can't imagine managing without the therapist's support and thinks that the therapist overestimates Mrs. H's abilities. She says that she sometimes feels like just leaving Anne at school instead of picking her up and that she does not have the courage to face the difficulties with Anne on her own.

When the therapist comments on what has just happened, Mrs. H starts to cry and says that everyone leaves her when she needs them, probably because she does not deserve to be helped. She goes on to say that her mother died when she was an adolescent and her husband left her when Anne was so difficult; now the therapist wants to leave her too, and she has no idea how she will manage on her own. When the therapist responds empathically about how anxious Mrs. H is about believing she can do things on her own this time, after having been let down so painfully, Mrs. H becomes calmer. The two of them spend some time thinking together about how Mrs. H's experiences of being left can leave her vulnerable when faced with endings. Mrs. H says that she realizes that she would be sad to not see the therapist but knows that she is able to manage on her own. She knows now that Anne's problems are not because she—Mrs. H—has done something wrong and that all she can do is do her best. And even when she does her best, she may not be able to fix everything. She knows all she can do is hang in there with Anne. The therapist suggests that they think together about how Mrs. H can best consolidate the changes that have taken place once they are no longer coming to therapy.

Deciding whether the parents are ready to end treatment should be guided in part by the ongoing assessment of their needs and developing strengths. As a general principle, the last few sessions should provide an opportunity to have an experience of an ending in which the parents and therapist can reflect on how to consolidate gains and maintain strengths that they have discovered but also, if needed, they can talk about painful past experiences of loss, separation, and individuation in the parents' lives.

Creating a narrative of the process of treatment in which the parents see themselves in the therapist's mind as agents of change for themselves and their child can help parents build on their strengths and maintain their sense of agency in the face of future challenges. Helping parents develop a balanced and realistic perception of themselves and their children, and understand what can be changed and what probably cannot and will have to be accepted, can help them overcome paralyzing feelings of guilt about being responsible for all of their child's difficulties. For example, if Anne continues to have behavioral difficulties at school, it can be a relief for Mrs. H to know that it is not the result of her being an inadequate parent and that nothing she can do will "make" Anne comply. For a mother overwhelmed by pressures from Anne's school, the child's distress, and her own concern, this can be of great benefit. When problems continue and the level of family need is more complex, home visits, with their ecological lens and wraparound interventions, can be particularly useful, especially to help parents maintain gains made in therapy.

CONCLUSION

The aim of working with parents in time-limited MBT–C is to help them develop their strengths and discover a reflective stance. This can help develop the kind of parent–child interactions in which children feel secure and understood, which in turn facilitates motivation, self-regulation, basic self-knowledge, and mentalizing. Many parents who come to consult may well have good reasons to approach therapists with a degree of uncertainty and mistrust, but when their vigilance relaxes in the context of a respectful relationship, they may be relieved and open up to new ways of understanding. As a result, parents are likely to show increased interest in the therapist's attempts to help them think about their child. Consequently, this stimulates and strengthens parents' capacity for reflective functioning.

8

MOVING TOWARD GOODBYE: ENDINGS IN TIME-LIMITED MBT–C

Because mentalization-based treatment for children (MBT–C) is a time-limited therapy, its ending is kept in mind from the start of the work. Using a calendar helps remind both the child and the therapist how many sessions have taken place and how many remain. Although some have argued that meaningful relationships cannot be established in short-term or time-limited psychotherapy, 3 to 6 months (which is the usual length of time-limited MBT–C) can be a significant period of time in a child's life, and we have found that children can form strong and lasting emotional attachments when working this way.

In this chapter, we present how the process of ending offers opportunities to explore ways to manage loss or goodbyes from a mentalizing perspective, but also the chance to consolidate what has been achieved, while giving the child (and parents) the confidence to generalize what they have learned into new settings. Being able to recognize when the therapy is not progressing, or

http://dx.doi.org/10.1037/0000028-009
Mentalization-Based Treatment for Children: A Time-Limited Approach, by N. Midgley, K. Ensink, K. Lindqvist, N. Malberg, and N. Muller

when it needs to continue further, is also essential. We explore the importance of assessing whether the child and the family are ready to end treatment or if additional (or alternative) interventions are needed. The chapter also illustrates how booster sessions can be used as part of MBT–C, after the therapy's ending, and explores how this may fit with a mentalizing focus.

INTRODUCING THE TIME-LIMITED NATURE OF THE WORK

Thinking about time and time limitation is not only an aspect of the last phase of therapy. The aim of every MBT–C therapeutic intervention is to encourage and increase the child's and the parents' ability to mentalize and regulate emotions in relationships to help them manage their difficulties beyond the end of therapy. Thus, the end is always in mind and is strongly linked to the process of assessment, as well as the goals and process of the treatment.

When we introduce the time-limited model to parents and children, it helps to explain what they can expect. A therapist might say the following:

> From our experience, and what we know from the research, the kind of issues that have brought you to seek help can often be sorted out with about 12 weekly sessions—in about three months. That doesn't necessarily mean that everything will be completely sorted out by that point, but we'd hope that we'll have made some real progress on the goals we set together and that you'd also have the skills and the confidence to continue getting help from each other and from the other important people in your lives. But each person, and each family, is different, so after about eight meetings, we'll sit down together and review how things are going. At that point, we can decide whether to stick with the original plan or to continue for a bit longer; or we may decide to think about whether there's something else that would be of help to you. I'll try and be as honest and open with you as I can in this process, and I'd really appreciate if you can be the same with me. If I am missing something or I get something wrong (which is always quite likely!), it makes my job easier if you can let me know, so that we can try and sort things out.

For children, it can be helpful to introduce the fixed number of sessions to give them a sense that there is a clear beginning and end. Parents can sometimes react in a way that suggests they think a limited number of sessions will never be enough, or they may feel that it is far too big a commitment, especially in terms of their own involvement. In the separate parent meetings, reflecting on these feelings can often open up valuable discussions regarding parents' feelings of helplessness, hopelessness, and their own insecurities as parents. If parents are concerned that the treatment may be too short for the difficulties the child is facing, we can ask them to think about whether they have had a brief relationship in their own lives that has been defining and important for them. Was there a teacher, a coach, a best friend, or a mentor who was in their life for a relatively brief time but whose influence they carry with them to this day? We can also reassure them that we will be meeting to review progress after the first eight sessions and that in cases where it is felt that more time is needed, this is something that can be discussed.

When discussing a parent's worry about the time limitation, the therapist should ideally focus on both the emotional content and give realistic information regarding the structure and length of the treatment. The therapist can be open about saying that, in his or her experience, many children profit from working within this time frame, but in some cases, time-limited work is not enough. Having the possibility in a service to make the choice to extend a therapy can be reassuring to both professionals and parents.

KEEPING ENDINGS IN MIND

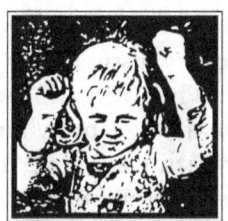 Mrs. H, Anne's mother, has arrived consistently late with Anne since their first appointment. Regardless of the therapist's attempts to stress the importance of punctuality and the impact it has when Anne has less time in her session, Mrs. H has not changed this pattern of behavior. She offers different excuses each time. After a particularly difficult session in which Anne showed her anger when the therapist stopped a game Anne started just as the session had come to an end, the therapists decide together that the parent therapist will address the issue with Mrs. H during the next parent session.

When they next meet, he reminds Mrs. H of Anne's behavior in the waiting room at the end of the previous session and points out that it is difficult for her to have so little time. He invites Mrs. H to imagine what this means for her daughter. Quite unapologetically, Mrs. H expresses her belief that the therapists could take a bit more time if they wanted to. The therapist says that he can appreciate that Mrs. H may feel like she's being told to do all the hard work and that other people, including the therapists, don't seem to offer much flexibility. (The therapist is mindful that Mrs. H and her husband are divorced.)

Mrs. H says, "Well, yes, I certainly don't get any help from my ex-husband in getting Anne to her sessions on time."

The therapist shows some sympathy, and Mrs. H visibly relaxes and becomes a little tearful. After a bit, the therapist goes back to the issue of punctuality and risks saying that perhaps, given all that has happened, Mrs. H wants to teach Anne something about people. Mrs. H smiles and says, "Like people leave you or let you down when you least expect it?" Then she adds, "It is never enough for her. . . ."

This vignette illustrates the multiple meanings of behavior around time and how important it is to invite parents to reflect and try to understand their child's experience from an inquisitive stance. Although Mrs. H initially indicates that the problem is the therapists' inflexibility, once the therapist responds in a nondefensive way, she is able to recognize that her stress is stopping her from being able to look at the meaning of being late from her daughter's perspective. We might say that Mrs. H is at first operating in a more teleological mode (i.e., thinking that the solution would be for the therapists to do something different by extending the length of the sessions). The therapist recognizes that the first task is to help Mrs. H feel understood and supported so that her capacity for mentalizing can come back online. In being able to speak to Mrs. H's own feelings of frustration and loneliness when confronted with the behavioral challenges of a 6-year-old without the support of a partner, the therapist shows a capacity to think about things from Mrs. H's perspective. Possibly due to shame, Mrs. H was not able to express these feelings openly, and instead they were expressed by disrupting Anne's time with her therapist. Perhaps fearing her child's and her own attachment to the therapist, she had found a way to stay emotionally distant by rendering the therapists ineffective and seemingly greedy with their time in her mind and that of her child. Once Mrs. H felt understood (and not judged), the therapist was able to help her get in touch with her daughter's experience of missing time with her therapist, and after this meeting, Mrs. H was more careful to bring Anne to session on time.

In time-limited work, the aspect of time is present in each session: keeping track of time, recording progress, and trying to keep the goals in mind. For children, working with the calendar makes the planning of the therapy visible (see Chapter 3) and is a reminder of the time-limited nature of the therapy. Children with separation anxiety, histories of loss or trauma, or attachment problems often find it difficult to end sessions (Gil & Crenshaw, 2016). As described in Chapter 2, we might come to understand this in the light of their attachment patterns and their mentalizing capacity.

The moment of saying goodbye at the end of a session is often an opportunity to learn about and support the child's capacity to mentalize. For example, some children run off immediately; others want to give the therapist a hug or even a kiss. Sometimes children feel so close to the therapist that they fantasize about them becoming a part of the family. Being sensitive to the meaning of the way a child says goodbye, or what the therapist feels when saying goodbye, and trying to use this information in therapy to explore the longings, wishes, or blank spots in a child's mind can help in understanding how the child deals with closeness and attachment needs. Even more important, it might open a dialogue about what the child misses or how she experiences the important people around them. Exploring what happens in the here and now between therapist and child and what kind of feelings you, as a therapist, are left with at the end of each session can give information about the implicit relational processes and can become an important basis for further therapeutic work.

DECIDING WHEN IT IS TIME TO STOP OR TO CARRY ON

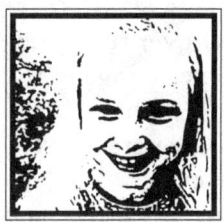

Belinda doesn't sit in a chair during the review session. Instead, she stands in a corner, playing with a plastic dog. She doesn't want to answer any questions. She seems to listen to her mother and the therapist but says only that she wants to go to her own session to play. When the parents and the therapist agree that she needs 12 more sessions, Belinda is pleased.

During the second review session, midway through the second block of 12 sessions, Belinda once more finds it hard to join the conversation, but this time she is willing to sit in a chair, pay attention to what everyone else is saying, and react to the conversation nonverbally. Her parents and the therapist again decide that she needs another 12 sessions, which will be the last set of 12. She seems better able to control her arousal level in this review session but still finds it difficult to contribute her own thoughts and feelings to the meeting.

In the final review session, during this last block of 12 sessions, Belinda sits in her chair and says to the therapist and her mother that she knows she is sometimes a "refusing horse" and sometimes a "wild horse" but that the horse has reins, and she can also be the jockey sitting on the horse with the reins in her hand. She sits in her chair proudly, as if sitting atop a horse, and everyone in the room agrees that Belinda is now in the right place to begin the process of ending therapy.

As described in Chapter 3, the therapist explains at the beginning of the treatment that after the first eight meetings, there will be a review session in which the parents, child, and therapist(s) look back over their work together so far and decide whether to move toward ending therapy or to continue with 12 more sessions, up to a maximum of three sets of 12 sessions. Alternatively, the therapist and family may decide that a different kind of intervention or support is needed.

The decision to stop or continue therapy depends on a number of factors:

- whether the problems that brought the child to therapy have diminished and the goals set by the family have been met, and whether the child, therapist, and family feel that continuing with therapy would help to further achieve this;
- whether the child has (re)gained a capacity to play, if this was inhibited, and to modulate and regulate her emotions (or use an adult's support in dyadic regulation to do so) in an age-appropriate way;
- the ability of both the parents and the child to mentalize in an effort to deal with misunderstandings and repair relationships when there are setbacks;
- clues provided by the quality of the calendar over time (e.g., on Belinda's calendar, shown in Figure 8.1, the change in the images she has drawn can be used to reflect on her experiences over time and, in this case, are a sign of her greater self-coherence and ownership of her narrative); and
- whether the family and wider social context are supportive, and the parents are able to provide the necessary emotional care for the child and the child is able to make use of this.

Deciding when to end a treatment is a challenging aspect of being a practitioner. Many of us are driven in part by our need to support and help; we may often believe that "something more can be done" (Fragkiadaki & Strauss, 2012). Sometimes ending therapy evokes strong feelings of loss, guilt, or inadequacy in the therapist, and sometimes of relief and freedom, especially when dealing with complex and challenging families or children. Some therapists, especially those not used to working in a time-limited way, can find it difficult to acknowledge that the therapy has a fixed length before

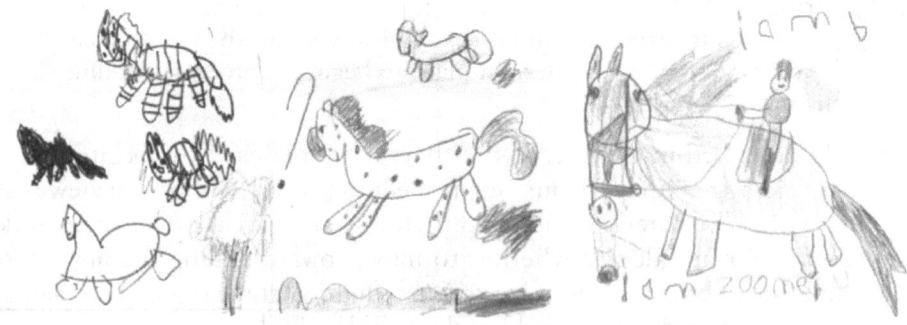

Figure 8.1. Belinda's calendar: Session 7, Session 19, and Session 31.

it even begins. Perhaps this makes the therapist reluctant to invest whole-heartedly in the therapy or allow a deep bond to develop. In these situations, supervision can be helpful to reflect on the therapist's ambivalent feelings and doubts about working in a time-limited frame or ending therapy. Therapists can use this information constructively to know whether there is something urgent that still needs to be addressed or to accept the limitations and frustrations of time-limited work, without depreciating the value it may have.

PREPARING THE CHILD AND PARENTS FOR THE REVIEW SESSION

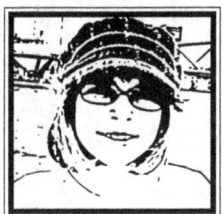

Ruth has now completed seven sessions of MBT–C. During this time, she has learned to show parts of herself, express herself more, and develop an understanding of "this is me from the outside, and this is me from the inside."

During the last few minutes of each session, the therapist invites Ruth to draw something on the calendar. In the first session, Ruth was hardly able to draw anything, tentatively drawing just three little lines. In the second session, she drew herself with open eyes, as if saying, "Yes, I can see you." After a few more sessions, Ruth spontaneously began to experiment with drawing faces and started expressing an understanding of how she sometimes feels things on the inside that she doesn't express on the outside. She realized that despite having severe emotional problems, she always seemed to smile at everyone rather than show her feelings.

Eventually, she took the colored pencils and wrote "inside/outside." An important theme in her therapy is that she doesn't feel seen by her foster parents. At the end of her fifth and sixth sessions, she put question marks on her drawings, as if to ask, "What do people see when they look at me?" She then seemed to start realizing that other people cannot know what she is feeling unless she can express something about it rather than pushing people away. In the last of these seven drawings, she showed her inner feelings, as if she was ready to look at her inside feelings and thoughts and was developing a sense of confidence about expressing them (Figure 8.2).

As part of their preparation for the review meeting, during their eighth meeting, Ruth and her therapist look back at the way she has created her calendar and use it as a way of reviewing what has happened so far in the therapy. The therapist is able to check out some of his own thoughts about Ruth's progress, and this opens up a discussion about whether they should be looking to end after 12 sessions, as they had

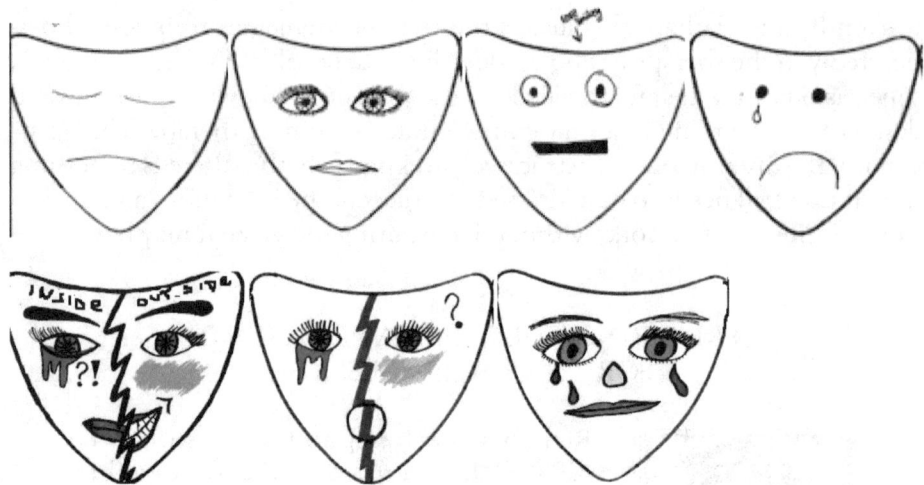

Figure 8.2. Ruth's calendar.

originally planned. They don't make any definite decision about this but agree to take some of what they were thinking about together into the review meeting with her foster parents and social worker.

The review session serves as an opportunity to solidify the child's sense of agency regarding the process of the therapy. Therefore, it is important to prepare for this session with the child. Sometimes the calendar can be a helpful tool in discussing the therapeutic progress. In the preceding example, the therapist reflected with Ruth on her drawings to clarify the meaning of the changes in them over time. Ruth could see that she was learning to trust others and started to understand that if she could express what she felt to others around her, then she could get something back from them in return. (The therapist noted to himself that this seemed to reflect an increase in trust, suggesting that Ruth would be able to continue to make use of other relationships to learn and grow, even if therapy ended.) The therapist asked her if she was willing to share these insights with her foster parents and social worker at the review meeting the following week, and she agreed to do so.

The review session often presents the challenge of having an open discussion while safeguarding the child's confidentiality. This can prove especially difficult when there are cultural beliefs regarding the (lack of) rights of children to their own privacy. Discussions about this with parents present an opportunity to explore the idea that the child is an individual with his or her own thoughts and feelings and private internal world, within the context of a specific cultural group (Gil & Drewes, 2005).

Preparing children for the review session and asking them what is OK to share and what is not is considered good practice and can help to build trust in the child that the therapist is considering things from his or her point of view. During this conversation, it is important to acknowledge external reality, for example, by letting the child know if there has been any contact with his or her school and whether the teacher has noticed any changes in the child's behavior.

In preparing for the review session with parents, they are usually asked what they have learned so far about themselves or about their child, which serves as a way to help the parents verbalize and consolidate their developing understanding of the child. They are also asked what they think they might need in the near future to be able to maintain the progress that has been made. Sometimes the therapist may be concerned that parents will not come back even if it might be necessary because they have concerns about appearing weak or having failed if they ask for additional help. It is important to explore whether there are feelings like this and what they mean to the parents because it is easier to end therapy when there is a reciprocal faith about letting each other go, knowing the therapist will be there if needed.

As part of these discussions, it can also be helpful to ask what the parents think should be shared with their child from their own meetings and what would not be appropriate to discuss. For some parents, this question can be a useful way to think about things from the child's perspective, which may illuminate what aspects of the parental situation may not be appropriate to share.

THE REVIEW MEETING

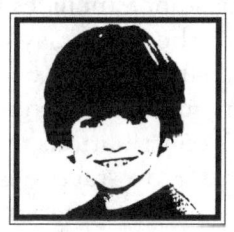 Mohammed, his father (Mr. D), and his father's partner (Ms. L) are present in the review session with their therapist. Mohammed looks anxious. Mr. D, who seems relaxed, smiles at Mohammed in a reassuring way. Ms. L is sitting silently but smiling. The therapist starts the session by reflecting on the fact that Mr. D and Ms. L seem more relaxed and able to reassure Mohammed. Ms. L nods. When asked why she nodded, she tells the therapist that she is very happy with how things are going. She feels Mohammed and his father have gotten over everything that happened with the car accident and things are beginning to be normal again. When asked what she means by "normal," she laughs and says, "A fish is not aware of the water in which he swims unless it is taken away from him." Everyone laughs in the room because of the way Ms. L has expressed her thoughts.

Mr. D explains they were not used to talking about what they feel but that he has learned so much about doing that with Mohammed, and this has helped him better understand his son. Mohammed is asked if he sees things in the same way. He nods. He is asked about the focus statement of their therapy: "Figuring out what will help you feel in control again." Mohammed says, "I am a fish, and I need water. Because of the accident, my bowl was broken—but now I know that I need water to feel happy." The therapist laughs and says that she can see that this is a family of poets! Then Mohammed, his father, and Ms. L talk together about what has been helpful in therapy and how things have changed for the better. There seems to be a strong, shared view that the work of therapy is coming to an end.

The central aim of the review session is to provide an opportunity to discuss the progress of the work to date and clarify the aims of the remainder of the intervention. As discussed in previous chapters, by the end of the review meeting, a decision is usually made about whether to move toward an ending, whether another set of 12 sessions is needed, or whether some other form of intervention may be required (e.g., parent–child therapy, family therapy). Going back to the goals that were set at the beginning of therapy helps remind everyone where things were at the beginning of the work, allowing each person to consider whether progress has been made (Law & Wolpert, 2014). In settings where other empirical measures of progress are used, these may also be consulted.

At the same time, this review session is a good opportunity to observe the parents' capacity to facilitate the child's participation while protecting him from information that may be hurtful or damaging. The preceding vignette illustrates how the atmosphere in a session can reflect the changes that have taken place. The therapists' mentalizing stance includes curiosity about the different perspectives the people in the room may have. Some young children may find it difficult to express their views because they have learned or have been instructed to listen quietly to the grown-ups in the room. In this context, the way the child's contributions regarding the ending of therapy are allowed and considered establishes the groundwork for any explicit mentalizing around issues of separation and loss. Furthermore, the ways in which the child and parents react to such a discussion can provide further information about their current reflective capacity.

Opportunities offered by the review session in time-limited MBT–C include the chance to

- reevaluate initial therapeutic goals in the context of current functioning,
- explore the meaning of the ending,

- provide an opportunity for the child and parents to express their unique perspectives regarding the process of psychotherapy in a secure environment where multiple perspectives are encouraged and respected,
- increase the child's and the parents' sense of ownership over the process of therapy, and
- practice communication about problems in a constructive way, together as a family.

In these review meetings, it is especially important to remember that information about the process can be shared, but the content of the child's or parents' therapy is confidential. Sometimes talking with the child about an upcoming session with the parents can be an opportunity for reflecting together, thinking about what would be helpful for a parent to know, from both the child's and the parents' perspective. The therapist can tell the child that the session is coming up and ask him if there is anything in particular he would want the therapist to tell or show the parents. The decision to end or continue therapy depends on how quickly the problems diminish and whether goals have been met; if not, do the child, family, and therapists think that continuing therapy could help to achieve these goals? Negotiating this decision is itself part of the work of promoting mentalization, exploring the situation from multiple perspectives, before making a final decision.

As part of the review process, it may be important to check in with the child's school regarding his or her progress. Information from this contact can be brought to the review meeting to share and reflect on in the context of the question "How are we doing in therapy and outside of it?" Parents and teachers (and therapists) can sometimes measure the success of a therapeutic intervention in very different ways. It can be challenging to bring these different viewpoints and agendas together, holding on to the value of what we have observed in therapy without assuming that we have a "truer" view than anyone else. As therapists, we only see the changes taking place inside the therapy setting and may have less perspective on how this relates to the way the child is managing in other contexts. Thus, the review session helps the therapist to see things "from the outside," and the therapist can help the parents and others involved in the child's life to see things "from the inside."

THE LAST PHASE OF THERAPY

Belinda arrives at her therapist's office. The therapist is aware that there are only two more sessions before their goodbye. Belinda is looking around the room and seems quite solemn. Her therapist notices her facial expres-

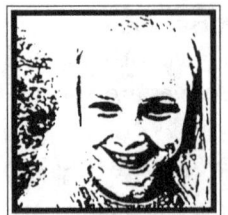

sion and says something about it: "You seem a bit lost as to what to do in here today. Did I get that right?"

Belinda smiles and replies, "I'm going to miss playing with the sand tray . . . and you."

"I'll miss you too, Belinda," her therapist responds.

Belinda begins to draw and tells her therapist that she is beginning dance classes next month. She also talks about a play date she has for the following week. The therapist comments that it is sad to say goodbye, but it is happy to think about all the new things she will be doing now that she feels stronger inside.

Once a decision has been made to move toward ending therapy, we may hope to see a shift regarding the role of therapy in the child's life. The child may gradually explore ways in which her external life feels safer now and may talk about ways in which her outside life will fill in the empty space left by the ending of therapy. Other children, however, will decide they "hate" both the therapy and the therapist, turning them into something useless and ineffective. All of these ways of managing the pain of separation and loss regarding ending therapy may reflect existing and remaining difficulties, but they may also represent opportunities to face such experiences in the context of a planned ending.

In general, the last few sessions, with both the parents and the child, should potentially provide the opportunity for

- a developmental experience of a meaningful goodbye;
- exploring experiences of loss in both the child's and the parents' lives;
- exploring issues of separation within the context of each person's family and larger culture; and
- thinking about gains and how to follow up and consolidate what has been learned in the context of treatment, with a particular focus on how the child and parents can make use of relationships in their daily life to support them.

Creating a narrative of the process of treatment with parents—one in which they can witness themselves as agents of change for themselves and their child—can prove an extremely powerful motivation for further change and strength in the context of current and future contextual stressors. In the same way, creating a balanced (strengths and weaknesses) profile of the parents, their child, and their relationship communicates to the parents a belief that they can be the "experts" going forward.

In MBT–C, the therapist may actively introduce some activity with the child that helps to prepare for the ending. Some therapists might want to create a small box for the child to take home after the last session, containing pictures and any other items the child and the therapist have created together. Others may create a song or a funny story about their therapeutic journey together. We can talk about other times when the child has said goodbye and connect these to the way she feels about ending therapy. Some therapists write an ending letter for the child in which they share some of their views on the work that they have done together. All of these can be important ways to mark the ending, although as therapists, we need to be careful not to force a "good" ending when the child may actually feel angry or hurt and need to express that in the way he leaves (Blake, 2008). In such cases, the therapist may have to allow the child to end therapy without the kind of positive feelings that Belinda expressed.

For children who have experienced multiple losses in their lives, this phase can prove extremely painful. The work of the therapist in such cases will include psychoeducation with parents or caregivers to understand behaviors that may emerge in response to the ending of treatment. In this way, while working with the school and the home, we increase the chance that these children will encounter adults who are trying to support and understand their challenging or puzzling behaviors as communication of their pain and fear, and not necessarily as defiance or being oppositional.

For other children with more internalizing tendencies, we might observe a withdrawn style of interaction and a general tendency toward avoidance as endings approach (Gil & Crenshaw, 2016). The challenge here is for the therapist to help these children explore and express their feelings about the ending. Many times, therapists find themselves facing a wall of avoidance as the final session approaches. Suddenly the symbolic play stops, and the child engages in mind-numbing activities. The therapist feels shut out. It may prove invaluable for the therapist to use those feelings to guide her or his ability to explore the child's experience.

In the final meetings with parents, it can be helpful to talk about how they can balance their focus on the child with their own self-care (e.g., by thinking about what gives them the energy to keeping going when life is stressful). This may take the form of asking for help within their network or simply recognizing when they need to take a break or get some fresh air. It may mean talking about how to stay open in relationships within and outside the family and avoiding harsh self-judgment or isolation. Sometimes we create a "first-aid kit" in the form of a list the therapist and parents write together describing what they have learned about managing challenging situations. This can help parents understand their difficulties in dealing with their child and knowing what the "banana peels" may be that they can expect to slip on. This helps convey the message that problems and setbacks will inevitably happen, but the parents now have increased resources to cope with them.

AFTER THE END OF THERAPY: "BOOSTER SESSIONS"

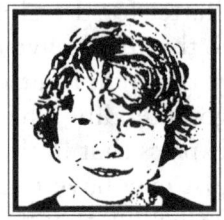

John's foster parents come back for a booster session 3 months after ending therapy. They enter the room with big smiles on their faces. The therapist comments on their relaxed appearance and asks them how things are going with them, John, and their family. Mrs. F answers that she is really happy. John is doing fine, and her earlier worries about whether therapy had been long enough are discussed. She had stopped working because of all the problems at home and is now thinking about applying for a new job. Mr. F is a man of few words, but he says, "I am really happy with our little chimpanzee in the house. I always wanted a son, and it really feels like he belongs with us now."

Once therapy has ended, we recommended offering *top-up* or *booster sessions* in MBT–C. This can be arranged in a number of ways, but the general aim is the same: Knowing that there is another meeting planned when the family and therapists will see each other again to talk about progress, or to identify ongoing or new difficulties, can contribute to a continued feeling of being kept in mind. The child or parents can ask themselves, "I wonder what the therapists will say about this when we talk in the booster session?" This can help them remember what they have learned in therapy and maintain a reflective and curious stance. It can also contribute to a sense of safety, reducing stress and anxiety or, if things have deteriorated, offer an opportunity to reconsider what kind of support the child and family may need.

One way of organizing this is to plan a booster session with a set date 3 to 12 months after the final therapy session. The appropriate length of time before the follow-up depends on the needs of the family and the outcome of treatment, and the time can be negotiated. When the therapist suspects he may need to plan for additional clinical interventions, the follow-up time may be shorter (sometimes even shorter than 3 months) than when working with families who do not report a lot of problems when therapy is ending.

An alternative approach to organizing the booster sessions, which leaves more responsibility with the family, is to use the *voucher model*. In this approach, the family is told that they have a certain number of "vouchers" (typically one to three) to use for booster sessions when needed. It is up to the child and family to decide when (or if) to use these, giving them greater freedom to reflect on what their needs are and to have more control over how they engage with services.

The choice of which of these two models to use may be based on what's possible for the therapists (e.g., whether you will be able to offer a booster session within a reasonable time if the family calls using the voucher model) but also on an assessment of the family's needs. This is something that can be discussed with the family when therapy is coming to an end and models the open-minded and collaborative approach that characterizes MBT–C. For high-functioning families with the ability for self-observation, the voucher model may be a good choice because it stimulates agency, leaving the responsibility to them to decide when they need help. Thinking about when to use the vouchers can promote mentalizing and self-observation in the family. For families who are unlikely to use the vouchers when needed, or who need more continuity, it may be more suitable to plan a date for a review or booster session before ending.

Sometimes it is most appropriate to have the entire booster session together with the child and the parents in the same room, but if two therapists have worked separately with the child and parents, they may want to have some time apart before they all come together. Especially for older children, this can help the family reflect together on their process and any obstacles they have encountered. The therapist can use the calendar to look back on the therapy with the child and find out how things have been going for them since they last met.

If things have been difficult since therapy ended, helping parents regain a mentalizing stance, as described in Chapter 7, is an important aim of the booster session. Sometimes parents come back to booster sessions urgently wishing to resume treatment. One way of handling this is to schedule a few sessions for the parents to discuss the pros and cons of reinitiating therapy, as well as to see whether it is possible to help them get back on track independently before planning further interventions with the child.

WHEN THERAPY ENDS UNEXPECTEDLY

There are many reasons endings may sometimes be abrupt or unplanned, although one of the advantages of time-limited work is that it tends to reduce the level of premature termination (Ogrodniczuk, Joyce, & Piper, 2005). Nevertheless, there will be times when, for a range of reasons, therapy has to stop before the planned ending. That does not mean that these endings cannot still be opportunities to validate and empathize with a difficult external reality that often renders both the therapist and the family feeling helpless and frustrated.

The most common reason children stop attending therapy abruptly is because parents decide to stop bringing them. Parents may say this is because they feel that the therapy isn't being helpful (or that it is making things worse) or that it is too great a burden to bring the child. Sometimes parents want to end treatment because they cannot take more time off from work, because other children in the family need their care, or for financial reasons. These concerns should always be taken seriously and the reality of external circumstances recognized. In some cases, such concerns can offer an important opportunity to explore something that has gone wrong and address misunderstandings.

However, when faced with a family that has determined that they cannot continue therapy, the therapist in MBT–C should attempt to manage some kind of planned ending, one that includes acknowledging the loss and saying goodbye. In this context, the goal is to have at least one session where the child is able to say goodbye and the parents are able to return without fear of retaliation and see that their wish to end treatment is understood and respected. Such situations can be difficult, especially when the therapist may feel angry about the child's therapy ending or think that the decision is a bad one. In these situations, the MBT–C therapist will try to acknowledge the external and internal realities and help verbalize other feelings associated with the process of saying goodbye.

Sometimes a child does not want to continue therapy because of a healthy desire to use the time to be at school or with friends, or simply to avoid the discomfort and pain emerging from the sessions. It is difficult for therapists to know when a child's desire to leave treatment should be discouraged or respected. Because the parents are regularly involved in treatment, the therapist can discuss with them the child's wish to stop. The therapist can also tell the child she really wants to understand and explore his wish to stop coming.

When a child is unable to commit to therapy but the problems are getting worse, it is necessary to consider whether the child needs more intensive therapy (e.g., day or inpatient treatment) or whether some other approach should be considered.

CONCLUSION

One of the key features of any time-limited approach to therapy is being mindful of endings from the start of the work. In this chapter, we have described how the therapist in MBT–C can work with endings, both throughout treatment and during its final phase. The process of endings is a time of consolidating therapeutic gains and internalizing the accomplishments in the context of saying goodbye (Novick & Novick, 2005). There is always more to do, but MBT–C aims to plant the seeds of curiosity and genuine empathy, providing enough "emotional oxygen" to both the child and parents that they can face the pleasures and challenges of life beyond therapy.

9

TIME-LIMITED MBT–C: A CASE STUDY

In this chapter, we present an account of a 24-session treatment (two blocks of 12 sessions) with Lulu, a 6-year-old girl who was adopted. We hope to illustrate the process of time-limited mentalization-based treatment for children (MBT–C) and show how the mentalizing frame and stance of the MBT–C therapists allow for a process of emotional coregulation, feedback, and developmental restoration to take place. This case illustrates the work with the child and the parents, as well as some of the interactions between the two therapists and their peer supervision that contributed to their work with the family.

REFERRAL AND INTAKE INFORMATION

Lulu was adopted from China at 2.5 years of age by a middle-aged couple with two older biological children. Lulu's parents, Mrs. and Mr. S, contacted the clinic, motivated by their feelings of exhaustion and helplessness in

http://dx.doi.org/10.1037/0000028-010
Mentalization-Based Treatment for Children: A Time-Limited Approach, by N. Midgley, K. Ensink, K. Lindqvist, N. Malberg, and N. Muller

parenting their two older children while adequately supporting their adopted child, who they felt tested them beyond their limits with her demands. During the first telephone contact with Mrs. S, she described Lulu as having frequent violent outbursts in which she seemed completely unreachable, followed by excessive clinging behavior toward her. Early in this conversation, Mrs. S began to cry, saying that she was at a loss as to how to manage Lulu.

ASSESSMENT SESSION WITH THE FAMILY

The clinical team decided that two therapists would work collaboratively with the family, one with the parents and one with Lulu. This was because the problems of the child and family appeared to be complex, and working with two therapists offered the possibility of sharing different perspectives and also sharing the responsibility and pressure that the initial referral suggested could be put on the therapist. After the initial meeting with the parents, both therapists invited the whole family to a joint assessment session. They had planned to begin by asking each of the family members to introduce the person sitting next to them. This proved difficult to do, as the family immediately started to display some of the difficulties that had brought them to therapy in the way they interacted, leading the therapists to realize that some flexibility was needed. The following is a description of the beginning of that initial meeting, from the perspective of the therapist who would later work with the parents.

> What first caught my attention was how striking Lulu's special position in the family was, as she demanded her mother's constant attention by pulling at her and whining, leaving no room for anyone else. The session started with everyone choosing a place to sit, and Lulu immediately demanded, "I want to sit next to mommy!" Both her sister (age 8) and her brother (age 9) also wanted to sit next to their mother, so what seemed like a common struggle ensued. When I curiously asked the mother what it was like for her to have all three children wanting to sit on her lap or close to her, she did not reply directly to me but explained to the other two children and myself that Lulu had missed so many "mama-hours." Because of this, she said, she had to give Lulu more attention, and she expected the other children to understand this and be sweet about it.
>
> The mother seemed to be under so much pressure that she couldn't join me in any reflection on the situation. Lulu's siblings looked furious with her, and it seemed to me that the situation was almost unbearable for them. I noticed their facial expressions and said that they looked angry, then checked whether my impression was correct. They started to tell me immediately that it was always like this. Lulu always wanted mama, but she was their mommy too! Mr. S explained that he tried to make up for

this imbalance in the family by taking the oldest two children out to play outside or for special activities, but everyone seemed to feel left alone, "on their own island." The older children seemed to agree.

To try to create some space for curiosity about each person's experience, the therapists talked with each other out loud during the session about how they experienced the atmosphere in the room. They especially noticed the interactions between the children, as they struggled to listen to each other's different perspectives. Both Lulu and her older brother seemed highly distractible and restless, moving around and not being able to sit in their chairs. Noticing this, the parent therapist spoke to her colleague directly and wondered whether it would be a good idea to shift the format of the session by engaging in something more active than the usual activity of choosing animals for the family members. The child therapist replied to her colleague by saying she had also noticed that the kids seemed to be having a hard time joining the interaction, and then checked with the family and asked whether they could try something. The children seemed intrigued and the parents relieved. The child therapist then noticed that the children were looking at the drums in the corner of the room. She wondered whether they could try and do a music exercise together. The children responded enthusiastically, and the child therapist smiled and replied in a playful and inviting way: "Then let the music begin!" The children's curiosity and attention had been activated. At this point, everyone took a percussion instrument.

Music exercises can be used to try to enhance attunement and to experience the difference between "me, you, and us together." The parent therapist played a rhythm, and everyone tried to join and imitate her. She tried to help the family harmonize by paying attention to each other and taking turns deciding the rhythm and direction of the music. She experimented with playing loud and soft, quick and slow. Then someone in the family was asked to play a rhythm, and the others followed. How does one follow? How does one lead? Who is followed in the family? The therapists paid attention to whether different family members could play a rhythm that could be followed by the others, or if they, for example, played something too difficult. Could they think about what others are able to do or not? Were they able to mentalize each other at an implicit level, by the way they engaged in this joint task?

What happened next surprised the mother and the children as Mr. S took the lead and was very present in playing the basic rhythm. When talking about this afterward, they explained to the therapists that this was a new experience for this family because Mrs. S had the leading role most of the time. The children seemed to be having fun together. The atmosphere in the room changed from one of hostility to one of cooperation and mutual regulation and attention. Lulu was able, in an age-appropriate manner, to show with her facial expressions her concern about not daring to take the lead:

When she was asked to play a rhythm, she said she didn't dare. The child therapist reflected on her age and how sometimes not being able to do the things her older siblings were able to do may feel frustrating. Lulu's siblings seemed to be able to listen to this and, when asked about it, gave examples of their own experiences when they were younger and felt frustrated or ashamed because they were not able to do things that others seemed to be able to do easily. During this exercise, the therapists were able to observe some of the strengths of this family, and they spoke openly about them. One noticed out loud how the older siblings seemed to, for a moment, see Lulu as an insecure little girl instead of a "monster" and how this seemed to have some effect on their interactions during the session. She continued, commenting that it seemed that Lulu's siblings were flexible, curious, and open to new ideas and behaviors. She observed that it was a good indicator of the way they had felt supported and thought about by their parents throughout development and was a potential protective factor for them and Lulu.

ASSESSMENT MEETINGS WITH THE PARENTS

During this first meeting, Lulu's parents told the therapist that they adopted Lulu out of their desire to give a home to a child in need, as they felt so blessed with their two biological children. They went on to describe how they were unprepared for and overwhelmed by Lulu's extreme rivalry and jealousy toward her two siblings. They were distressed by her "hoarding" behavior and her tendency to steal things from her siblings and other children. They were concerned that Lulu had a negative self-image and was very isolated with no friends in school or in the neighborhood. Furthermore, they described how she was often controlling and insensitive toward other children at school as well as her siblings; this contributed to her becoming unpopular and being rejected by her peers and caused conflict with her siblings.

The meeting with Lulu's parents conveyed the frustration, helplessness, and loneliness they experienced in dealing with their 6-year-old daughter while also trying to taking care of the needs of their other two children. The parent therapist sought to validate and normalize the parents' feelings by speaking of what she imagined was their desire for a happy family as well as how their sadness and frustration with the current situation were understandable and not unusual. She also shared her experience regarding the process of adaptation that adoptive parents commonly go through. In addition, the therapist tried to impart some realistic hope by emphasizing that Lulu was still young and developing; she focused on some of Lulu's strengths and those of the family, such as the parents' real interest and curiosity about Lulu's behavior and how her early experience might have influenced the way she was now.

The therapist had videotaped the family session, so at this point, she invited both parents to look at the first 5 minutes of it and share their thoughts and feelings about what had happened. She asked them to look at the faces of the children and invited them to comment on what they might have been feeling or thinking. The parents were able to reflect about what it meant for their two other children that Lulu got more "mama-hours" and thought about how this might have affected family dynamics. Mrs. S reflected on her reasons for feeling that she needed to be constantly available for Lulu. She commented that she had experienced the adoption as a huge and important responsibility to take on, and how she desperately wanted to make Lulu happy so that she could feel the adoption was successful. However, at the same time, she felt guilty for what she felt at times amounted to "borderline neglect" of her biological children because she felt consumed by Lulu's emotional and other needs. Mr. S referred to Lulu as "the queen of the house," who completely controlled the family routines and schedule.

Mrs. S concluded by saying that she felt exhausted, and Mr. S added that although he could see how demanding this was for his wife, he could not help feeling left out. When they felt overwhelmed by these feelings, it was difficult to reflect and mentalize. Despite this, when feeling supported and thought about by the therapist, they could begin to explore the needs and wishes behind their children's behaviors. At these moments, their capacity for explicit mentalizing was high. They were able to reflect on the feelings of exclusion their biological children likely felt but also accept the therapist's attempts to normalize the fact that sibling rivalry is common in most families. This opened the door to an emerging balance between emotions and cognition, and new ideas for ways to support the children emerged in the conversation.

At the same time, both parents were able to reflect on Lulu's incapacity to accept the normal frustrations of having to share her parents with the two other children. Perhaps, the therapist said, Lulu feels like she isn't quite a full member of the family and therefore needs constant reassurance that this is her "forever family." Mr. S reflected on the possibility of Lulu having that feeling not only at home but also at school, where she possibly felt different as an adopted child, who also looked different from the other children because of her ethnic background. The therapist invited the parents to think about ways in which the family could support Lulu in feeling less like "a lonely island" and instead try to get the whole family to return to feeling like they all lived together on the same island.

The therapist and Lulu's parents tried to think of various ways to understand Lulu's anger, which was often expressed in unexpected and inadequate ways. The aim was not to find the "real" meaning of her behavior but to introduce the idea that the same behavior (anger) could be understood in many ways.

To support their curiosity about Lulu's mind, the therapist asked the parents about her early development. Not much information had been given to them about Lulu's early life and family history when they adopted her. Mr. and Mrs. S were told that she had been abandoned by her biological parents at a market and then taken to a private orphanage where several children lived under the care of one woman. At the time of the adoption, Lulu was overweight, which made Mr. and Mrs. S suspect that the children were given food as a source of comfort and to keep them quiet. In the early stages after the adoption, Lulu had severe aggressive outbursts, and she seemed to be unable to connect with other children; she also seemed unable to develop a normal eating pattern.

It is often helpful to think about the parents' own relational history. This can be an aid in assessing their reflective functioning as well as an opportunity to explore how their own past relationships influence how they cope with and respond to their children's behaviors. Lulu's father said that he was an only child, and he reflected on how this could be linked to his difficulties managing the liveliness and conflicts of his now larger family, with three children always begging for attention. Mrs. S, on the other hand, had grown up in a larger family with four siblings and therefore was used to dealing with conflict and chaos. Mr. S even said that he sometimes had the feeling that Mrs. S sometimes thought that the chaos in their family was a normal state. Together they could reflect on how their different backgrounds influenced their perspective on the current situation and also the way they understood and communicated with each other about it.

Regardless of all the frustration both parents felt, they exhibited a kind and generous demeanor when speaking of all their children, and Lulu in particular. They also showed a great deal of curiosity as well as a capacity to respond to the therapists' playful comments and invitations to reflect about themselves as parents. All of these characteristics helped the therapists to come up with a preliminary impression of the parents' reflective functioning as quite well developed. At the end of the parent assessment, the therapist asked them about their needs and what they wished would be the goals of the treatment. The parents said they wanted to focus on thinking of ways they could promote a healthier atmosphere for their three children and work toward feeling more unified as a family, supporting their children to express themselves while respecting each other.

The therapists concluded this session by encouraging Lulu's parents to introduce activities in which the three children could play and have fun together while supporting each other. The aim was to help Lulu feel connected in a positive way to her brother and sister, while feeling safe enough to experiment, learning how to ask for help, and feeling like she belonged. The parents decided to buy a video game console with three controllers for the family for Christmas. They also decided to start going to the local bowling alley on Sundays.

ASSESSMENT MEETINGS WITH THE CHILD

The following is the therapist's description of the beginning of her first assessment session with Lulu.

> It was not easy to establish rapport with Lulu. She seemed to reject invitations to mentalize and was resistant to name anything that troubled her; she did not seem open to any contact (verbal or nonverbal) with me at the beginning. She started the assessment by sitting in a corner with her back to me. I wondered if she was concerned for her safety, worried that I could turn out to be someone who could hurt or betray her. I decided to let her know that I could wait. I smiled and played casually with some sand in my hand as I observed her explore the room quietly but curiously. I would name some of the things she was looking at and made some simple comments such as, "Hmm . . . yes, those are my cars. Some are fast and some are slow." She began to smile shyly.

The therapist noted that Lulu presented as hypervigilant and very restless, much more so than would be expected for a child her age. As a result, her ability to play seemed inhibited. However, she could recognize and name emotions when prompted, which suggested that some of the building blocks of mentalizing were in place. When presented a chart with faces, she was able to identify and name most of the emotions, but she seemed unable to think of times and situations when she felt sad or angry and didn't seem aware of her own emotions as they emerged in interaction with the therapist in the session. For example, when the therapist asked her if she could give an example of things that made her sad or angry or think of a time when she felt these feelings, she couldn't, and even though she became quite angry with the therapist during some points in the session, it seemed like she was entirely unaware of this. When the therapist asked about the change in her face and wondered whether she was maybe feeling a little angry, Lulu shrugged and rejected this idea, saying that she was not and saying in a categorical and authoritative tone that angry feelings were not a problem for her. During the subsequent assessment sessions, the therapist noticed that Lulu did not seem to feel comfortable in her body: She carried her hand stiffly; was always hungry and wanting to eat during the session; and presented as very tense, especially when her sense of safety seemed threatened by the therapist's words or actions, which often seemed to be the case.

The therapist introduced the *family constellation exercise*, in which Lulu was asked to choose shells representing her family. Lulu chose three shells for her three mothers, explaining in a matter-of-fact way that she had a birth mother in China, a mother in China who looked after her in the orphanage, and her current mother in this country. The therapist asked her where she wanted to place each of these "mother-shells." She didn't know. Lulu wanted all three shells near to her shell. Meanwhile, the shells of the other two children in the family had to lie in a corner of the room; she didn't want to share the table with them. She chose only one "father shell," representing her adoptive father. When asked to say something about how it felt to create this story, she looked at the therapist without answering, as if the question was not meant for her or did not make sense to her.

Lulu struggled to settle on playing with anything in particular. She touched everything in the room in a restless way, repeatedly wanting to go out of the room and run in the corridor. It seemed that rather than being hyperaroused and reactive to external stimuli, Lulu was driven more by an inner sense of unease that was probably amplified rather than contained by being in the room with a person with whom she had not yet established a relationship of trust. The therapist, after reflecting on the context, decided to focus first on the fact that being with someone that she did not know might be stressful. The therapist said that she thought Lulu was showing her how difficult it was for her to be in the room, in the clinic, with someone she did not know or trust. Once Lulu seemed a bit more regulated, the therapist wondered if she could help her show her discomfort and mixed feelings she had about being in a new place with someone she did not know by creating something like a drawing or maybe by making some music. Lulu liked to draw and made a drawing of a beautiful flower, still under the ground, saying that it was the national flower of her adoptive country. After this, Lulu drew an airplane. The therapist casually commented on the pictures, saying it seemed like the little flower was still underground waiting to become a beautiful flower after flying to this new place in a plane.

SHARING THE ASSESSMENT AND DEVELOPING A FOCUS FORMULATION

On the basis of her individual meetings and a range of other standardized assessment procedures and questionnaires, it appeared that Lulu met many of the criteria for reactive attachment disorder. She also had symptoms of attention-deficit/hyperactivity disorder, and the child therapist discussed with her colleagues whether these symptoms could be part of the attachment problems or might be influenced neurologically by aspects unknown to the adoptive parents, such as fetal alcohol syndrome. The child therapist considered how the duration and severity of the traumatic losses in her life might be playing a role in the current problems. The fact that Lulu exhibited a growing attachment toward her adoptive parents (especially in wanting to cuddle, looking for affection, and asking for comfort from Mrs. S when she was upset), rather than looking for affection from others indiscriminately, seemed to be evidence of her resilience. It seemed that she could potentially make use of an MBT–C intervention, even if the focus was likely to be on helping her to establish some of the building blocks of mentalizing, rather than on the use of explicit mentalizing per se. The parents showed increasing insight in the family dynamics after only three assessment sessions, giving the clinical team the impression that it was likely they would also profit from further MBT. During the feedback session, both therapists spoke to Lulu and her parents about time-limited MBT–C. They provided the family with a general explanation of MBT–C and the rationale behind it, as well as how they felt this approach related to their family and specifically to Lulu's needs. The family accepted, and after establishing a basic social contract around the structure of treatment (day, time, frequency), the idea of a focus formulation was introduced as the first step in the process of intervention itself.

When trying to look for a focus formulation with Lulu and her parents, Lulu still did not say much. She gave the impression that she mostly wanted to be left alone, and she still didn't express any hopes or wishes about getting help. It occurred to the therapist that this seemed to be a common relational pattern for her where she pulled back and retreated from relationships rather than sharing her feelings, wishes, or ideas, perhaps because she had little experience doing so. On the basis of Lulu's behavior during the assessment, the child therapist had formulated an impression that Lulu thought of the world as unsafe, and she had little sense that adults could be trusted and attuned to her, or that they might be willing to see and hear her. It seemed to the therapist that, in response to her passivity, adults tried to take control to support her, but Lulu interpreted this as them not acknowledging her wishes and needs, strengthening her belief that adults were not interested in what she thought or felt.

Lulu's parents were pleased with the drawing of the flower when they saw it, and commented that Lulu too was like a beautiful little flower. Lulu responded by angrily saying that she wasn't a flower at all! It seemed as if she felt mocked and could not trust that her parents were genuinely complimenting her, seeing her this way and loving her despite her "thorny parts." The parents responded to this in a playful but serious way, saying that maybe Lulu was a caterpillar, always wanting to eat, often wrapped up in her own cocoon of anger, fear, or sadness, not being able to make contact with them when she needed them most, but that they thought that there was a wonderful colorful butterfly inside of her. They also expressed their hope that the therapy could help her become this beautiful butterfly, who could learn how to handle her big, angry feelings and practice playing with others and feeling more connected, finally feeling like she could leave the cocoon. There was a feeling of confidence and openness among the parents, Lulu, and the therapist. The therapist experienced this as both helpful and hopeful. The parents explained to Lulu that they also needed to learn more about how to be good parents for all their children. The parents and the therapist proposed together that the focus formulation for the therapy could be "caterpillar on a journey." Lulu was OK with this and even offered a little smile.

THE BEGINNING PHASE

During the first MBT–C session, the therapist and Lulu started by creating something that was linked to the agreed-on focus formulation as a way to further establish the focus and increasing Lulu's ownership of it. Together they made a clay caterpillar. While working with the clay, Lulu made angry faces. The therapist observed Lulu's body language, facial expression, and moments of greater tension, trying to get a better understanding of this nonverbal communication. The therapist mentioned in a casual and playful way that she noticed how Lulu was really good at following instructions when working with the clay, but that she was not sure that Lulu was really enjoying it and that Lulu's body and face seemed to be saying that. She checked with Lulu if she was getting it right, but Lulu ignored her, seemingly disconnected from both the therapist and herself. Toward the end of the first session, Lulu suddenly took a stuffed monkey, smashed it against the wall, and said with a different tone of voice, "You have to die!" She looked at the therapist in a challenging way as if asking, "What do you have to say about that?" The therapist got the sense that this was the first instance of a genuine feeling and action Lulu had exhibited. She said, "Monkey, I have no idea what you have done, but it seems to me that Lulu does not like you and wants you to disappear." Then, shifting her attention to Lulu, she said, "I sure would like to understand why you have such big feelings and want Monkey to die!" Lulu's body and face relaxed, as if the therapist had managed to make contact with her (possibly by speaking about the feelings a toy may have) followed by a direct inquisitive acknowledgment, said in a nonjudgmental, curious tone of voice, of the emotional experience Lulu was expressing.

After this session, the therapist decided to work with Lulu more physically, trying to give her space to follow her impulses and express herself in a physical way, allowing her to feel free to express her "big feelings." It felt as if a more physical focus could help Lulu develop the building blocks of mentalizing, such as joint attention and a level of affect regulation. So the therapist set up a special corner in the playroom with mattresses, pillows, curtains, kangaroo balls, boxing material, and other materials, inviting both motoric and sensory exploration. Lulu engaged with these materials enthusiastically but constantly tested the boundaries in the room—her own and those of the therapist. For example, one rule in the playroom was that they weren't allowed to walk in that corner with their shoes on, but Lulu completely refused to take off her shoes during the beginning phase. Furthermore, she started each session by climbing up a big pile of mattresses, trying to sit on top or glide away or in between them. The therapist found herself put in the position of reminding Lulu constantly that she had to keep her safe in the room and that Lulu therefore needed to come down from the pile. When observing Lulu, it seemed like she didn't care about herself with her reckless and accident-prone behavior. She often wanted to run out of the room as she had tried to do before, and the therapist firmly reminded her that they had agreed on staying in the room during their session. When in session with Lulu, the therapist tried to name what she thought was Lulu's longing to test her physical boundaries as well as the capacity of the therapist to keep her safe, while simultaneously keeping her in mind and not taking over the activity.

During team supervision the therapist "marked the task" as reflecting on how she could balance keeping Lulu safe in the room without turning into a police officer. The supervisory team members were curious about the therapist's own feelings when this was happening, and she shared her annoyance and frustration regarding this matter and reported feeling drawn toward coercive behavioral strategies to stop the defiant adventures of her patient. As she spoke, the therapist realized how difficult it was to keep mentalizing herself when being constantly challenged. She felt annoyed and anxious about Lulu's behavior. The therapeutic team then invited the therapist to imagine Lulu's experience. What could she be saying or asking with her behavior? The therapist thought Lulu's question was something like, "What do you do when I am in danger? Do you look after me? Do you care about me at all?" The MBT–C team reflected on the sense that Lulu was operating at a prementalizing level, looking for constant evidence from the therapist that she could keep her safe, would respond predictably, and have the capacity to survive her attempts at destruction. It was not difficult to understand how the therapist felt drawn in to the same behavioral rather than mentalizing stance, wanting to take physical action. In "returning to task," the therapist reflected that it probably was important for Lulu to see that she would actively intervene to keep Lulu safe but that she needed to remember Lulu was probably operating in a prementalizing mode because of her levels of anxiety and relational distrust; keeping this in mind would help her as a therapist to better manage the demands Lulu put on her.

During the sessions of this middle phase of the therapy, Lulu and her MBT–C therapist were trying to create a place where they could be together, where it felt safe enough to experiment, and where Lulu was in control but aware that she was looked after and kept safe and could begin to build trust in the therapist as someone who was interested not only in how she behaved but also in what was going on inside of her. Lulu's therapist would closely follow her in her movements while reflecting out loud on her own experience of Lulu's behavior. For example, she spoke about how she felt afraid that Lulu might fall, and she wondered what it was like for Lulu when she took these physical risks? When the therapist made these comments, Lulu would increasingly stop her play and listen. She became more present, and this was evident in her body posture, level of activity, and willingness to meet her therapist half way. Often her therapist would verbally track the sequence of events in the session and reflect on her own increased anxiety or capacity to feel more relaxed in relation to Lulu's behaviors and responses. It seemed that Lulu was feeling helped and increased feelings of agency and positive self image were starting to emerge. The therapist got the sense that Lulu started feeling and knowing: "I can influence the situation, my feelings are important, I am worth noticing and getting attention, my behavior has an effect on others."

In the following sessions, Lulu repeatedly killed the monkey in different ways—slapping him, riding over him with a huge kangaroo ball—screaming and saying he had to die. Her therapist observed and commented on what was going on, simply narrating and accepting Lulu's anger. The therapist thought that this allowed Lulu to experience herself as a physical agent, expressing anger and destructiveness toward the monkey in a safe and contained environment with the supportive presence of the therapist. She tried to help Lulu by narrating what she observed, linking it to what she thought might be going on inside her; it seemed important to Lulu that she could use her whole body to destroy the monkey. It was as if she were expressing a profound rage that lived inside her, and the therapist thought that what seemed most important was for Lulu to be able to express this in a relationship and have the experience that it could be tolerated, not reacted to as if it were real in the same way as if she were actually murdering the monkey. It could be viewed as an expression of her internal reality, and it was OK to *pretend* to kill the monkey and express herself in this way.

The therapist tried to remain nonjudgmental about her playing out such a murderous scene. At times she took on the role of the monkey, trying to express what she thought its feelings might be: "Aw, this hurts. Wow I can feel the pain. I am afraid—she is trying to destroy me. She wants me to die, but I don't understand why." In this way, the therapist attempted to label the emotions she thought the monkey would have to help Lulu find the words and create representations of her emotions, as she understood Lulu's play. Lulu ignored this. The therapist then changed her tone and tried to match Lulu's affective tone of excitement by mirroring her expression, as if the therapist were the television reporter of an important match: "Yes, what power you have! You are so strong." The therapist was trying to establish an environment of regulation and emotional feedback to promote mutuality while encouraging agency. She attempted this by trying to mirror Lulu's play in a marked and contingent way and by sharing her reactions in a direct manner using words but also her nonverbal communications in the here and now. All these can be thought about as the building blocks for the development of more explicit mentalizing capacities.

Working with children who express aggression often has an impact on the therapist's own mentalizing capacity. Peer supervision is extremely helpful in this context. This was certainly the case for Lulu's therapist who, in meetings with her team, expressed how anxious she felt witnessing Lulu's aggression in "killing" the monkey. At times, she said, she had difficulties thinking and staying in the here and now in the therapy room, as she felt concerned that she was not doing enough for Lulu and her family. The parent therapist then shared with the team that Lulu's parents were reporting an improvement in Lulu's capacity to contain her aggression at home and school. This indication that they were on track seemed to help the child therapist to restore faith in the therapeutic process, helping her stay present and think when confronted with Lulu's aggressive behaviors. In addition, the therapist had the impression that Lulu was playing out something around the experience of rejection and the hatred she felt for this scared and distressed part of herself; this was not simply a repetitive expression of cruelty and sadism.

After about five sessions, Lulu took the monkey and laid him down with her own teddy bear, putting a little blanket on top of them. The therapist asked the teddy bear, "What happened? Lulu seems different today. She is so gentle and careful."

Lulu picked up on the therapist's question and answered with a deep, teddy bear voice, "Yes, I told her that maybe the monkey is tired today, and so am I. So we need a day off."

The therapist thanked the teddy bear for explaining and asked how it could tell the monkey was tired. Lulu answered, "No idea." She then wanted to lift the foam rubber blocks and asked the therapist to time how many seconds it took her to move the blocks from one side of the room to the other. The therapist felt there was more contact between her and Lulu and was happy with this brief conversation with the teddy bear. Lulu now seemed to tolerate the therapist looking at her; she was answering simple questions and even asked her to be part of her play by timing the activity. The therapist continued to work on this new joint focus of attention by giving words to what she observed Lulu doing and, when possible, checking what she thought and asking for clarification and encouraging elaboration. She responded positively when Lulu displayed efforts to establish boundaries, both mentally and physically, between her and the therapist by making nonjudgmental comments. In this way, the therapist tried to help Lulu focus her attention on her physical experiences and help her be more attentive to what was happening inside her: "Your face turned red . . . what do you think is happening to you? This exercise seems to make you warm. You are out of breath, do you notice that? You are very quick and strong!" The therapist tried to validate her ideas and enjoy them with her.

The therapist was surprised by Lulu's attempts to test her strength despite her small frame. In peer supervision, she told her colleagues about how Lulu was moving the blocks. Her colleague shared an association she had, that it seemed as if Lulu was moving her two worlds, her homeland and her adoptive one, in a super-fast way. Hearing the different perspectives of colleagues helped the therapist try to keep mentalizing about what might have happened in the sessions, knowing these associations, interpretations, or hypotheses could help in trying to better understand Lulu's actions, when she so often lacked words to describe her experiences. The implicit and explicit mentalizing of the therapist in and after the sessions seemed to have a huge impact on the therapeutic process with Lulu.

During this phase of therapy, there was a focus on Lulu's sense of self-agency, with an emphasis on connecting her inner and outer worlds, her body and mind. Lulu responded positively to this and seemed to begin to enjoy contact with the therapist more and more, moving away from simply engaging in a repetitive physical activity where she moved blocks from one side of the room to another, which seemed to have a self-soothing and protective function. She reacted to the therapist's encouragement and seemed pleased by her enthusiasm about her physical strength. After exercising, her therapist encouraged her to stop and relax, beginning to introduce a focus on affect regulation. One exercise that really relaxed Lulu was blowing bubbles, an activity the therapist introduced to help Lulu become able to regulate her breathing and focus on something that made her feel calm. Being able to create the beautiful bubbles and watch them float away seemed to give Lulu a sense of calmness and control that she all too seldom felt. The therapist commented on the bubble-blowing feeling and said that Lulu looked as if she was able to deal with anything. She marked the feeling by mirroring Lulu's calm, in-control, and slightly blissful look as she felt that Lulu needed some mirroring of herself in this positive state.

At this point, the monkey was no longer thrown away at the end of each session, but Lulu put him in a corner, sitting with the other stuffed animals, and told him she would be back next time. These comments made the therapist think that Lulu was developing a sense of herself and her relationship with the therapist as something that would endure over time. She now trusted that they would meet again and that the relationship would endure the time away from each other. At the same time, it seemed as if she was now taking on a more caring role in relation to the rejected monkey part of herself that she previously seemed to have such hateful feelings toward.

At the beginning of their work together, the therapist felt that Lulu had little sense of continuity and predictability, and therefore the therapist used the calendar to help with this, talking to Lulu about how they were going to meet next week and how many sessions they had left, as well as looking back at previous sessions while Lulu was filling in the calendar. From initially seeming quite uninterested in these conversations, as time passed Lulu started taking more interest when the therapist talked about this, and after a while, she could make comments on previous and coming sessions as well. Then Lulu began to take the initiative by playing games she had seen on TV. One of her favorites was a quiz for children where they had to answer questions to test their knowledge while hanging on a climbing wall, testing their physical endurance at the same time. Lulu explained that she loved this quiz show and hoped one day to be on it. The therapist asked her what made her like it so much, and Lulu answered that she wanted to be "strong in her head and in her arms." This was new, as she was articulating and communicating something about her self and what she wanted. In addition, this was the first time she made any attempt to connect the world in the therapy room with the outside world. She continued to challenge herself physically, asking the therapist to count how many seconds she could hang on the door frame. Lulu pushed beyond her physical limits: Her muscles trembled, and her hands were red, but as usual, she did not really seem to connect with her physical sensations or use them to guide her actions. The therapist validated her longing, spoke about how she seemed to need to feel strong and in control, and focused on her urge to go far. After playing like this for a few sessions, it seemed like Lulu was able to connect her bodily sensations, feelings, and expressions a little bit more, stopping earlier when feeling her arms starting to tremble, still expressing how strong she was, with a certain sense of pride.

WORK WITH LULU'S PARENTS

During treatment, the parent therapist worked in parallel with Lulu's parents. She started by explaining how the therapy with Lulu would be working and explored their thoughts and feelings regarding the process of the individual therapy. Lulu's mother expressed her concerns regarding Lulu's delight in provoking the cats at home by trying to squeeze them or pull their tails and wondered if this was an early sign that Lulu lacked empathy and the capacity to care for others. Lulu had told her mom about the killing of the stuffed monkey in therapy, and Mrs. S expressed serious worry that Lulu hadn't developed a conscience. She felt anxious and believed she was failing as a mother or that Lulu's "damage" was so deep that nothing they could do would "fix" it. Lulu's father, however, reported that he found Lulu less aggressive at home since the therapy had started. He reflected on the possibility that the start of her life may have been painful but that she now was feeling safe to express these feelings in the treatment. The fact that they didn't know much about Lulu's first period of life was very frustrating for both parents. The therapist tried to help them reflect on what Lulu was trying to communicate with her behavior. They started to think together about this implicit information, and both parents started to consider other possible explanations for the things that Lulu sometimes did or said. Furthermore, the therapist explained about disorganized attachment, which was helpful for both parents because it helped them to feel that there was some sense to their daughter's behavior, even if it seemed as if it was nonsensical at times. Mr. and Mrs. S were asked to observe and try to notice shifts in their behavior and to try to do the same for Lulu. Where possible, they were also encouraged to help give words to some of the feelings that Lulu might be experiencing at home, but doing so in a tentative way that did not assume they knew for sure what Lulu was feeling. The therapist thought this might help Lulu develop her capacity to recognize feelings in herself and others, while seeing that her parents respected and understood that her mind and experiences were separate from theirs.

Later in therapy, as a result of Lulu's newfound interest in physical expression, her parents enrolled her in gymnastics at school, and she seemed to have a talent for this. At the same time, the therapist had asked both parents to keep a reflective log, which resulted in them realizing that Lulu's outbursts often occurred when Mrs. S wasn't home. This made the therapist and parents reflect together on the interactions between Mr. S and Lulu. Mr. S felt that he had difficulties showing his love for Lulu because she seemed so clear about preferring Mrs. S; this made him feel redundant and insecure. The therapist invited both parents to consider whether there might be other reasons Lulu behaved like this, and this led them to wonder whether Lulu had ever experienced two adults caring for her together and what experience she had had of male caregivers. This led Mr. S to consider whether his relationship to Lulu was perhaps more important than he had realized. When asked about what he liked about Lulu, he had a hard time coming up with something, which shocked him. The therapist asked him to think of something he had liked doing himself with his parents when he was young. He remembered that he loved to go to soccer games with his father and decided to take Lulu alone to the next match, as he sometimes did with the other children.

During this phase of the MBT–C intervention, the therapist also made contact with the school. Lulu's teacher had questions about how she could stay better attuned to Lulu. They had a conversation where the therapist shared some information about attachment disorders, and together they explored possible classroom interventions. Specifically, the therapist encouraged Lulu's teacher to pay more attention to her own reactions to Lulu and to help Lulu express more about her feelings by being curious and presenting her with tentative explanations and helping her notice and become curious about the feelings of others. The teacher and therapist agreed to stay in touch, mostly by e-mail, establishing in this way an environment of collaboration in which the valuable role of both teachers and therapist was acknowledged.

REVIEW SESSION

During the review session, which took place after eight sessions, Lulu said that she liked attending therapy and wished to continue. Both parents were surprised to hear Lulu state her feelings so clearly. Although there had not been a great deal of change in the rating of the behavior checklist that had been used when Lulu started therapy, her parents said that they noticed her being more at ease at home and less angry. They also felt that they had made some progress in their own goal of creating a healthier atmosphere between their three children and commented that their other two children were no longer feeling as if Lulu took up all of their parents' attention. The parent therapist asked what they thought their other children might have said if they had been there today. (The parents had decided not to bring them to the review meeting.) Mrs. S thought they would have agreed that their parents were being more careful about not making them feel Lulu got all the attention and that this had actually improved their relationships with their adoptive sister. Mr. S noted that the siblings may experience the situation in different ways, reflecting on the perspectives of each one of them. The parent therapist noted how carefully they were thinking about the children's respective experiences and wondered what other people who knew them might say about how Lulu was doing. Mrs. S said that the school had told them that she was not trying to eat all the time as before and that she seemed a bit more relaxed, even if she had not yet managed to make any close friends and could still be quite a handful in class. The child therapist asked Lulu about school, and she said that she didn't like it when she had to sit outside the classroom on her own.

Having spent some time reviewing how things were, both the therapists and Mr. and Mrs. S felt that Lulu needed to consolidate her new strengths because they were not yet sure that Lulu was able to generalize what she was learning in therapy to other key relationships (e.g., with teachers and peers). Lulu was a girl with limited epistemic trust, something the therapist had thought about from the start of the treatment when considering whether a single block of 12 sessions would be sufficient. At the end of the meeting, there was therefore a mutual decision to go on for another 12 sessions, after the first block of 12 sessions came to an end.

MIDDLE PHASE OF THERAPY

After the first phase, Lulu started to engage more in pretend play. She had a fantasy where she was a queen of "the other world," and she and her teddy bear could not feel any pain. Up until then, she had been very much in a teleological or psychic equivalence mode, where her feelings could become "too real" and overwhelming. However, she started to experiment, first in a controlling way, telling the therapist exactly what to do. Gradually she began to accept the therapist's invitations to "be together" where she tried to stay in contact with Lulu in the play, following her lead while retaining her own boundaries regarding safety, wondering, often out loud, about what Lulu was thinking and feeling.

The therapist felt that Lulu remained quite rigidly stuck in either fantasy or reality, with no evidence of age-appropriate flexibility. For example, she started to make a throne using rubber blocks, wanting to be the queen far above everyone and in control. This was somewhat hazardous, and repeatedly Lulu nearly fell from her throne of blocks, testing the attentiveness of the therapist. Lulu seemed to be playing out her own game, with the therapist allowed to be only a spectator. She rejected or ignored any attempts by the therapist to engage in the play and did not respond to suggestions or questions from her. She seemed unable to accommodate the perspective of others in her play and showed limited explicit mentalizing, especially for considering the thoughts and feelings of the other. However, Lulu was also beginning to express her own feelings in a more contained fashion, with the support of her therapist who tried to provide a safe context. Gradually, play started becoming more reciprocal, which allowed the therapist to find a balance between keeping it both challenging and playful.

A few sessions later, Lulu's play took a turn when she decided she wanted to take the queen's role and wanted the therapist to play a baby lying on the ground with a nappy on. She said that she wanted to "dump" the baby. When the therapist asked her what "dumping" meant, Lulu shrugged her shoulders and ran around repeating the word loudly, over and over again. The therapist noted that Lulu's feelings had suddenly gotten big, and she wondered what had happened. She asked her if they could stop and think together for a minute. Guided by her awareness of how difficult it is to think when you are in a high level of emotional and bodily arousal, the therapist did not try to immediately review what had happened. Instead, she invited Lulu to follow her in "pretending to blow bubbles," a variation on really blowing bubbles that had relaxed Lulu in earlier sessions but was now operating at a more symbolic level. This calmed Lulu down, and when she was calmer, she wanted to reengage in pretend play with the therapist. In the story, the therapist was lying on the ground being a baby with a nappy on, getting "dumped." Lulu tried to cover the therapist with several blankets, roll balls over her, and put the foam rubber blocks around her, hitting her with a soft ball. However, Lulu's level of regulation had improved, and so had her capacity to stay in contact with the therapist. She could now accept the therapist's limits when she said that she did not want Lulu to roll the kangaroo ball over her head. The therapist tried to keep talking to Lulu with different tones of voices: a voice of the baby being dumped, a voice of herself as the therapist setting limits, a voice of the therapist empathically subtitling what Lulu seemed to be doing. Considering Lulu's tendency to be overwhelmed by fantasy or play, slipping into the prementalizing mode of psychic equivalence, the therapist thought of this as a way of further helping Lulu stay in the play by marking what was fantasy and reality in a concrete way with different voices.

When making notes about the session after Lulu had gone, the child therapist noted how this session literally took her breath away. She felt Lulu's fierceness and power in wanting to harm the baby and imagined that she was in part expressing her hatred of this abandoned part of herself. Writing this down helped her to mentalize Lulu's experience of feeling "dumped" as an abandoned child, and she understood this as a way for the child to actively manage the narrative of her early life and feel in control of it by being the one dumping the baby. She thought that it might be important for her to share this with the parent therapist because she might want to let the parents know that Lulu was now actively exploring her own experience of being adopted and invite them to pay attention to whether there were any differences in how she was at home. She felt that sharing with the parents thoughts and feelings about the process of the child therapy could be helpful, although she was careful not to go in too much detail about what had been said or done, in order to respect Lulu's privacy and right to confidentiality.

At the next session, Lulu seemed reluctant to talk about what had happened in the previous week. Guided by her awareness that it might help Lulu to make the implicit more explicit and to construct a coherent narrative, the therapist decided to draw a little book trying to make up a story about a little caterpillar on a journey, arriving in an upside-down world full of monkeys and meeting a queen who was strong and fierce. She had made some drawings that she and Lulu could finish together, trying to make it a book in process. The therapist had put all her creativity in the little book, feeling that she wanted to give Lulu the best she had, motivated by the strong feelings she had felt in her role as the dumped baby, and thinking how this was probably a taste of the rejection that Lulu herself might have felt as a baby. This was so intense that the therapist found herself powerfully hoping that the therapy could help Lulu to feel seen, mentalized, and helped to overcome her destructive feelings, and finally be able to mourn.

The therapist presented the book to Lulu, who refused to even look beyond the first page. Instead, Lulu became very dysregulated, running around the room and trying to escape out into the corridor. She screamed, "I hate caterpillars! I hate your book, and I hate you!" and she began to kick and push the therapist, who struggled to continue mentalizing, not understanding this strong reaction, while feeling under physical attack by this very angry little girl. The therapist lowered her body, took Lulu's hands and said she could tell she had made a serious mistake, even if she did not yet understand what she had done wrong. Lulu did not seem to respond much to what the therapist said, but the latter's body posture and calm voice seemed to have a calming effect on her. The therapist reflected to herself that Lulu needed help with very basic self-regulation before they could think together about what had happened. She tried to remain calm and signaled to Lulu with her hands and her tone of voice that she needed to simmer down. She told Lulu it was OK to be angry but that at the same time, she could not act out in ways that would be unsafe for the therapist or Lulu herself.

The therapist was taken by surprise when, all of a sudden, Lulu collapsed on the cushions in the room and began to cry. The therapist kept talking to her with a soothing, low tone of voice, trying to keep in contact with her. Then Lulu suddenly stood up, took a pin from the bulletin board, and jabbed herself, saying, "Bad Lulu!" Her therapist stopped her and reminded her that she would always keep her safe but that she could see she felt something inside and was looking for ways to communicate what she felt. In the moment, it was difficult for the therapist to make sense of what had happened, but she understood this as Lulu regressing to a teleological mode, where only an action (stabbing herself) could be used to manage strong feeling states. However, at this point, the priority was to help Lulu become less dysregulated, so the therapist simply spoke to her in a soothing, empathic way, expressing her own view that she didn't think Lulu was bad but acknowledging that she seemed upset and felt misunderstood. The therapist continued that it was sometimes so difficult to understand each other and to know what was the right thing to do—like today, where she had clearly gotten something wrong and was really sorry.

In peer supervision, the therapist was angry with herself and expressed her sense that she had crossed a line in trying to explicitly connect the child's play and fantasy too early, knowing that she couldn't yet integrate them, but wanting to give her a special homemade book. However, there was a space for mentalizing that led to reparation after what she felt had been a painful rupture between the child and the therapist. Once the group had helped the therapist regain her own mentalizing capacity, she was able to think together with her colleagues about what might have been the reason for Lulu's powerful reaction. Although at the time, everything happened too fast for her to think it through and make sense of it, the therapist now had a sense that Lulu felt betrayed by her, perhaps because Lulu had started to trust her as a helpful and respectful facilitator of her emerging sense of agency and of herself, and that creating and giving the book to Lulu had somehow surprised and overwhelmed her. The book that the therapist had meant to further validate Lulu's story (the therapist's intention) was experienced as somehow doing the opposite. Or it might have been that by making the play too tangible, realistic, and concrete by putting it in a book, Lulu connected for the first time in an explicit way with her own life experiences, which seemed too unbearable to handle. The therapist realized in peer supervision that her own mentalizing capacity had been influenced by her desire to rescue this child, feeling so sorry for her and at the same time feeling powerless to take away Lulu's pain. In a similar way to the parents, who sometimes felt let down and helpless when faced with Lulu's inability to use their containing and loving efforts, the therapist had reacted to the same feeling of helplessness by providing something concrete too quickly, acting in teleological mode. During meetings with the parents, this episode was used to explore the feelings Lulu's parents experienced, including the shame they felt. The therapist's use of self (mentalizing her own experience in the session) while sharing with the parent therapist, who communicated to the parents her colleagues' experience, seemed to help these parents to further mentalize their shame and anger toward their child and reflect on the impact it had on their parenting. The parents told the therapists that "a miracle" had happened after Lulu's emotional outburst in her last session: Lulu was relaxed, playing with the construction material with her brother, and eating well for the first time in many months.

THE ENDING PHASE

After the difficult session with the caterpillar story, the therapist invited Lulu's mother to join the next session because she felt this might help restore a sense of safety in the room. A conversation ensued in which Mrs. S, Lulu, and the therapist could talk about the relationship between Lulu and her therapist. Lulu could tell the therapist that she was neither a caterpillar nor a queen. She was just Lulu. The therapist apologized once more, and Lulu seemed calm and listening. She said she didn't want to play today and asked if they could draw something together as they had done at the start of the therapy. The therapist agreed, and Mrs. S sat by the side and watched for a while, until Lulu turned to her and said, "You can go and see Mrs. A [the parent therapist] now."

Once the paper and materials were out, Lulu wanted to paint a panda, an important symbol in China. She asked the therapist if she could help her by drawing the outline so she could color it (see Figure 9.1). Afterward, she wanted to glue a little monkey in the picture. It seemed to the therapist that Lulu wanted to make her own little story with her own symbols in it, being the one to choose and decide. She expressed again that she didn't want a caterpillar on her painting, as she didn't like them. Lulu started to explicitly talk about what she liked, what she wanted, and things that had happened at school or at home.

The creation of Lulu's painted story took a few sessions. The painting expanded: She wanted more paper glued to the first piece. During these sessions, the therapist felt surprised as she observed an emerging sense of self-agency and Lulu's verbalization of feelings. The therapeutic work with Lulu now felt as if it had moved to a different level, where the creation of the story about the panda made it possible to explore a wide range of thoughts and feelings. Neither Lulu nor the therapist linked the story back to her own experiences explicitly, but there was a strong sense that they were working

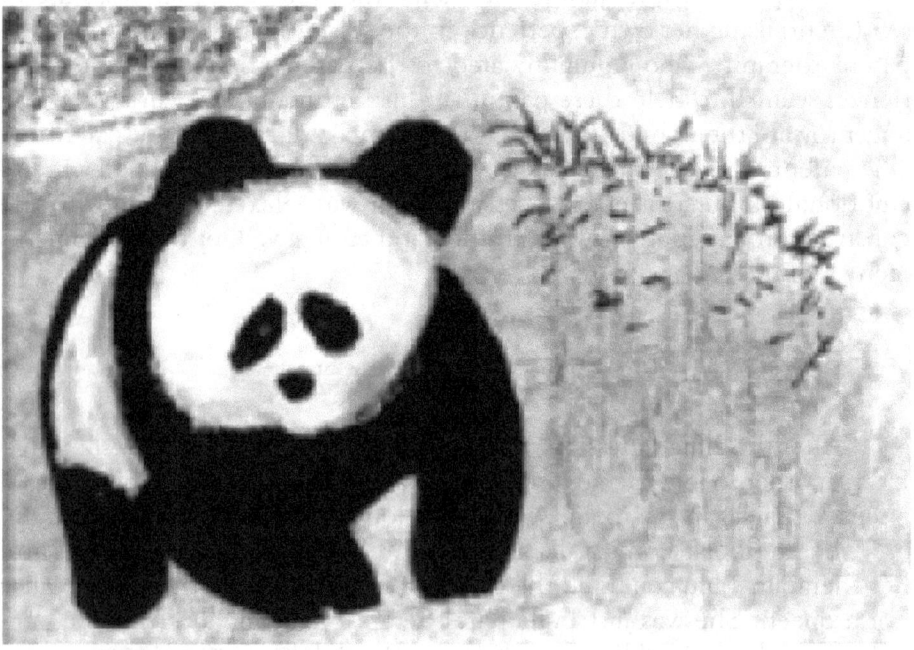

Figure 9.1. Lulu's drawing of a panda.

on something that was emotionally significant, and the act of creation had a powerful internal drive to it. For the first time, the therapist was able to make use of techniques to promote explicit mentalizing, such as mentalizing about the characters and relationships in the play context. Drawing on a popular television series that she had seen, Lulu told the story of a panda who went to a new zoo in another country, having new adventures, seeking something he had lost, looking for new friends, and looking for food. The therapist's role was to support the telling of this story, sometimes drawing figures and taking on specific roles, and sometimes asking questions about the thoughts, fantasies, wishes, and feelings of the main characters. At times, the panda met other characters, and the therapist and Lulu were able to use these narratives to explore a range of feelings and experiences, including new themes that seemed to play an important role in her life now. These included curiosity and difficulties about playing together, sharing, wanting to belong, and wanting to be special, even as an "outsider."

THE SECOND REVIEW SESSION AND WORKING TOWARD AN ENDING

The therapists, parents, and Lulu met for a second review session after a total of 20 sessions. By this stage, there was a noticeable improvement on the behavior checklist, especially for items related to behavior with peers. More important, the parents reported that Lulu seemed to allow herself to enjoy the intimacy with her parents and siblings. At school, her teacher had become fond of Lulu. In therapy, Lulu had managed to repair her sense of safety with her therapist, who wanted to help her understand herself in this new world. The world of adults seemed to have begun to feel safe and helpful for Lulu, and this increased her capacity to manage her "big feelings" and, most important, try to understand them with the support of those who loved her. It was agreed by all that the therapy should come to an end after the second block of 12 sessions was over.

During the last phase of contact with the parents, they reported seeing changes in Lulu that made them happy and hopeful. Mr. S had gone to a soccer match with her. Lulu had enjoyed it but at the same time had been a bit overwhelmed by the huge stadium, searching for his hand all the time and sitting on his lap during the match. For the first time, he said, he felt that he was her father, feeling how she could relax against his body, feeling the warmth of sitting there with his daughter, being able to protect her and offer her an exciting new experience. The situation had changed for the rest of the family, as well. Mrs. S felt less exhausted and freer to be the mother of all three of her children. At school, Lulu started to make friends with other children and was invited to a birthday party for the first time. There were no longer violent outbursts, and parents and teacher continued to reinforce Lulu's attempts to calm down and tried to always be curious and "wait it out" with Lulu instead of trying to fix things right away.

The therapist discussed with Lulu whether they could think of something to do together in the last sessions and wondered out loud if the focus formulation "caterpillar on a journey" should be a part of these last sessions. She remembered aloud what had happened before when she had got it wrong and brought in the book about the caterpillar. Lulu answered that she didn't like the caterpillar, but she liked butterflies. She found a wooden picture frame in the therapist's cupboard with space for two pictures. She chose to paint this frame during the last two sessions and brought a picture of herself and her (adoptive) mother to the last session to put in the frame. The therapist asked why she wanted her mother in the frame with her. Lulu answered that she loved her mother very much and although she had had two other mothers somewhere in China, this mother was going to stay! In the last session, the therapist gave Lulu a postcard, with a little text about how she had seen Lulu change during the sessions, about how much she had learned in working with Lulu, and saying that she would never forget her. Lulu gave the therapist a beautiful drawing in a somewhat tough, but at the same time shy, way.

CONCLUSION

MBT–C treatment provided Lulu with a safe space where she could experience and express her anger, fear, and sadness while feeling supported. During the first phase of therapy (the first block of 12 sessions), the focus was primarily on building the foundations for mentalizing, with a particular emphasis on joint attention and affect regulation. Much of the work was carried out at a physical level, helping Lulu to feel "at home" in her body and the therapist offering an experience of contingent and marked mirroring. Midway through this first phase, the therapist felt that she and Lulu had a real "moment of meeting" after a significant rupture, and that after this, the work had been able to move to another level, where the focus could be on more explicit mentalizing and the creation of a narrative around Lulu's early experiences of loss. The parent therapist worked on supporting the system by offering a containing and nonjudgmental space to Lulu's parents. Furthermore, the parallel collaboration between both therapists, while being supported by the therapeutic team, provided a mentalizing space when confronted with the feelings of helplessness in response to the child's anger and the parents' frustration. Finally, by starting the therapeutic work with a focus on attention regulation, followed by an emphasis on affect regulation, Lulu's mentalizing capacity began to emerge and develop, which helped her regulate her emotions and increase her attention control, in turn helping her to further develop her explicit mentalizing capacity. By the end of the 24 sessions, Lulu and her family had gained enough from the therapy to be able to continue the work themselves, but with an understanding that at later stages of her development, as new issues might emerge for Lulu, they would have the option to come back to the service, knowing it was a space where they could feel supported, heard, and cared for.

CONCLUSION: LOOKING BACK AND LOOKING FORWARD

In this book, we have outlined a particular way of working with children and their families that we consider to be representative of time-limited mentalization-based treatment for children (MBT–C). In Part I, we introduced mentalizing as a theoretical model and proposed a framework for the normal development of mentalization during childhood, as well as failures of mentalization and our understanding of how these may be linked to psychological difficulties for which children and families frequently seek professional help. In Part II, we outlined the structure and aims of time-limited MBT–C, describing the therapist's mentalizing stance and the process of assessment, then presenting elements of the direct work with the child and the techniques and approaches this involves. We also described a mentalization-based framework for working with parents, before moving toward goodbye and endings in time-limited MBT–C. Finally, we presented a case study in which we illustrated the approach typically used in MBT–C, starting with the assessment of

http://dx.doi.org/10.1037/0000028-011
Mentalization-Based Treatment for Children: A Time-Limited Approach, by N. Midgley, K. Ensink, K. Lindqvist, N. Malberg, and N. Muller

the strengths and difficulties of Lulu and her family and the conceptualization of the problem from a mentalization perspective, through the beginning of treatment, to the review sessions, and finally to the end of treatment.

In writing this book, we have tried to crystallize the key notions and presented the time-limited MBT–C model that has emerged over the years as we have practiced it and that we consider is faithful to the concepts and approaches of MBT as developed by Bateman, Fonagy, and their collaborators. Some readers may feel that much of what is described in this book is close to what they are already doing when working with children in therapy. If this is the case, perhaps our work offers an opportunity to reflect on the extent to which mentalization is a common factor in psychotherapy. As we noted at the outset, MBT is in many ways an integrative therapy that draws on elements from a number of existing therapies and aims to enhance our focus on one element (mentalizing) that may well be a common factor in a number of evidence-based interventions (e.g., Goodman, Midgley, & Schneider, 2016).

In this Conclusion, we look backward to touch briefly on how the work presented here originated, and then look forward and consider what remains to be done. We hope this book will serve as a guide but also inspire others to adapt and further develop this basic approach to best address the needs of children and families when working in various contexts.

LOOKING BACK

As set out in the introduction of this book, mentalization based treatment can be seen as emerging out of a fruitful dialogue that took place among clinicians trying to develop more effective treatments for borderline personality disorder; philosophers exploring the concept of 'theory of mind'; and developmental researchers investigating attachment and, in particular, the question of the intergenerational transmission of attachment patterns.

However, as we argued in the introduction to this book, clinical work with children can be seen as having played an additional role in the development of MBT and should not only be seen as an "adaptation" of MBT to a new clinical field. As early as 1965, Anna Freud recognized that using traditional child analytic techniques for treating children with "developmental disturbances" was likely to be unsuccessful and called for new developments in the technique of child analysis (Freud, 1965). She gave her clinical staff at the Hampstead Child Therapy Clinic (renamed the Anna Freud Centre after her death) considerable freedom to experiment with different ways of working with these complex cases, resulting in the ground-breaking papers on technique with borderline children written by her colleagues Rosenfeld and Sprince (1965) in the early 1960s. Following Anna Freud's death in 1982, Fonagy, Moran, Bleiberg, Target, and others continued this strand of work, demonstrating how the lack of a fully formed theory of mind can underlie the kind of developmental disturbances that are so common in referrals to child mental health services, and offered the outlines of a clinical approach to child treatment under the umbrella term of *psychodynamic developmental therapy* (Fonagy & Target, 1996a).

In their 1998 paper on the changing aims of child analysis, Fonagy and Target focused on three elements in particular which they suggested were of particular importance in psychodynamic developmental therapy: (a) a capacity for playfulness, (b) a focus on enhancing reflective functioning, and (c) the need to work in the transference. All three of these elements are elaborated on in the book edited by Anne Hurry in 1998, *Psychoanalysis and Developmental Therapy*, which along with Stanley Greenspan's work on developmentally based psychotherapy (Greenspan, 1997) and Verheugt-Pleiter et al.'s work on mentalization-informed psychoanalytic psychotherapy (Verheugt-Pleiter, Zevalkink, & Schmeets, 2008; Zevalkink, Verheugt-Pleiter, & Fonagy, 2012), is perhaps the most complete early articulation of what a mentalization-based, psychoanalytic developmental child therapy could look like. Other elements that have significantly influenced the model of time-limited MBT–C set out in this book include: (a) the important work on parental mentalizing and maternal mind-mindedness undertaken by Arietta Slade, Elizabeth Meins, and others; (b) the developmental research by academics such as Csibra and Gergely (2009), which has thrown light on the emergence of social cognition and mentalizing in early and middle childhood; and (c) the creative adaptations of MBT for use with families (Asen and Fonagy, 2012a, 2012b; Keaveny et al., 2012).

LOOKING FORWARD

For the authors of this book, coming from five countries has challenged us to clarify and present a model of MBT–C that represents what is common to our work across our diverse settings, in addition to our individual perspectives of what MBT–C is or should be. This international collaboration has enriched our model of MBT–C in many important ways—through learning from each other and accommodating each other's perspectives, as well as considering cultural variations that we tend to take for granted until we realize that the norms and practices differ by country and tradition. For example, a sand tray is a common component of the playroom in some countries but not in others. There may also be cultural differences in how therapists may position themselves in relation to the families they work with, how they prefer to be addressed, and how relatively formal and neutral versus informal and "friendly" they may be with the families. Working together to author this book has helped us to become more aware of these differences and enriched the way each of us thinks about the way we practice and what we teach.

We believe that the guiding light for working with children and families, as well as training students and future therapists to do this work, is a respect for and interest in psychological experience, together with a curiosity about the way that people's thoughts and feelings inform how they behave.

This brings us to the training and conditions that we think are necessary to successfully work in this way. Emerging from a psychodynamic tradition, we hope that this way of working can be practiced by child therapists with a wide range of interests and specialties. Those wishing to do so would need a basic training in conducting psychotherapy with children and families but would also benefit from specific training in the practice and techniques of MBT–C, with a particular focus on working with the mentalizing stance. This is also the case with MBT for adults, where core therapeutic expertise is complemented by MBT-specific training. Furthermore, we consider that ongoing supervision, especially in work with challenging cases, is necessary to provide the best service and to continue to develop as therapists. Supervision is not simply another tool in a therapist's toolbox; it can play a central role in helping the child therapist maintain the mentalizing stance, especially when faced with the emotional challenges that are an inevitable part of therapeutic work with children and parents. So, too, especially when working in the public sector, it can be difficult to maintain a mentalizing approach without the support of the institution itself in terms of the value given to feeling, thinking, and talking about the children in therapy. As resources for public services become increasingly stretched and fail to allow for the "safe uncertainty" (Mason, 1993) that is so central to mentalizing therapy, there is a risk of entering into a prementalizing mode of thinking characterized by the need to "do something" or to lose our curiosity about the experience of self and others.

Although we have described a basic MBT–C approach, including principles and techniques that we believe are applicable clinically to the treatment of children presenting with many types of psychological difficulties, additional research is necessary to further our experience with the model. In addition to the creative work that is always necessary to adapt a model or approach in a way that is optimal for individual patients, it is certain that looking forward, additional effort in a number of areas is important. First, time-limited MBT–C should be adapted to optimize it for specific populations.

For example, for children with serious externalizing difficulties, MBT–C may need to be adapted to address more specifically the difficulties and needs of these children and their families. This will require elaborating a model of the key mentalizing problems and associated interventions to specifically address these difficulties (see Hoffman, Rice, & Prout, 2016). Similarly, further work is needed to adapt MBT–C for children with developmental disorders, such as those on the autistic spectrum or those with intellectual disabilities, based on a clear understanding of the range of mentalizing difficulties that contribute to and underlie these difficulties and with interventions especially elaborated to address them. Furthermore, the basic MBT–C treatment model presented in this book was developed to be generally applicable in clinical practice to treat children with various presenting difficulties, including children with depression and traumatized children; however, in the context of presenting a general treatment approach, it has not been possible to comprehensively address all the nuances to be considered for any specific population.

Second, work is needed at the level of evaluating time-limited MBT–C and collecting the empirical evidence to confirm whether this approach is effective. Although practice-based evidence and preliminary evaluation look promising (Thorén, Pertoft Nemirovski, & Lindqvist, 2016) and the logic of focusing on promoting mentalization in children and parents has considerable empirical support, there is an urgent need for well-designed evaluations of the approach to better understand "what works for whom, under what circumstances, and why." As always, when it comes to something as vital as addressing the mental health needs of children and families, much work remains, but we hope that readers of this book will have sensed our passion and excitement about this model and find inspiration in the ideas we have shared.

APPENDIX: MEASURES OF REFLECTIVE FUNCTIONING IN CHILDREN AND PARENTS

The following clinical research assessments have been developed and validated to assess mentalization for research purposes, but they are also widely used (and adapted) by clinicians because of their clinical utility. To meet the standards of being able to publish using these assessments in peer-reviewed journals, trainings are provided by the developers to ensure that coders are fully familiar with the concepts and able to reliably code the interviews. However, the full interviews, as well as short versions or individual questions taken from them, are widely integrated into clinical assessments. There is little doubt that it is ideal and also stimulating to enroll in full training where the background of the development of the measures, the theoretical principles and assumptions on which they are based, and the nuances of coding and interpretation are explained. Such training is essential when using the measures for research purposes. But even without such training, familiarity with these measures may be useful for clinicians.

1. ASSESSMENT OF PARENTAL REFLECTIVE FUNCTIONING

Manuals

Slade, A., Aber, J. L., Bresgi, I., Berger, B., & Kaplan, M. (2004). *The Parent Development Interview—Revised*. Unpublished manuscript, The City University of New York, New York, NY.

Slade, A., Bernbach, E., Grienenberger, J., Levy, D., & Locker, A. (2004). *Addendum to Fonagy, Target, Steele, and Steele Reflective Functioning Scoring Manual for use with the Parent Development Interview*. Unpublished manuscript, The City University of New York, New York, NY.

Validation Article

Slade, A., Grienenberger, J., Bernbach, E., Levy, D., & Locker, A. (2005). Maternal reflective functioning, attachment, and the transmission gap: A preliminary study. *Attachment & Human Development, 7*, 283–298. http://dx.doi.org/10.1080/14616730500245880

Contact person: Arietta Slade (http://www.pditraininginstitute.com)

2. ASSESSMENT OF REFLECTIVE FUNCTIONING REGARDING TRAUMA

Manual

Berthelot, N., Ensink, K., Normandin, L., & Fonagy, P. (2015). *Trauma Reflective Functioning coding manual*. Unpublished manuscript, Laval University, Québec, Canada.

Validation Articles

Berthelot, N., Ensink, K., Bernazzani, O., Normandin, L., Luyten, P., & Fonagy, P. (2015). Intergenerational transmission of attachment in abused and neglected mothers: The role of trauma-specific reflective functioning. *Infant Mental Health Journal*, 36, 200–212. http://dx.doi.org/10.1002/imhj.21499

Ensink, K., Berthelot, N., Bernazzani, O., Normandin, L., & Fonagy, P. (2014). Another step closer to measuring the ghosts in the nursery: Preliminary validation of the Trauma Reflective Functioning Scale. *Frontiers in Psychology*, 5, 1471. http://dx.doi.org/10.3389/fpsyg.2014.01471

Contact persons: Nicolas Berthelot (Nicolas.Berthelot@uqtr.ca) and Karin Ensink (Karin.Ensink@psy.ulaval.ca)

3. ASSESSMENT OF REFLECTIVE PARENTING IN INTERACTION

Manual

Normandin, L., Leroux, A., Terradas, M. M., Fonagy, P. & Ensink, K. (2015). *Reflective Parenting Assessment coding manual*. Unpublished manuscript, Laval University, Québec, Canada.

Validation Article

Ensink, K., Leroux, A., Normandin, L., Biberdzic, M., & Fonagy, P. (in press). Assessing reflective parenting in interaction with school-aged children. *Journal of Personality Assessment*.

Contact Person: Lina Normandin (Lina.Normandin@psy.ulaval.ca) and Karin Ensink (Karin.Ensink@psy.ulaval.ca)

4. ASSESSMENT OF CHILD AND ADOLESCENT MENTALIZATION/REFLECTIVE FUNCTIONING

Manual

Ensink, K., Target, M., Oandasan, C., & Duval, J. (2015). *Child Reflective Functioning Scale scoring manual: For application to the child attachment interview*. Unpublished manuscript, Anna Freud Centre/University College London, London, England.

Validation Article

Ensink, K., Normandin, L., Target, M., Fonagy, P., Sabourin, S., & Berthelot, N. (2015). Mentalization in children and mothers in the context of trauma: An initial study of the validity of the Child Reflective Functioning Scale. *The British Journal of Developmental Psychology, 6*, 1–15.

Contact person: Karin Ensink (Karin.Ensink@psy.ulaval.ca)

5. ASSESSMENT OF CHILD ATTACHMENT

Manual

Target, M., Fonagy, P., Shmueli-Goetz, Y., Datta, A., & Schneider, T. (1999). *The Child Attachment Interview (CAI) protocol*. London, England: University College London.

Validation Article

Shmueli-Goetz, Y., Target, M., Fonagy, P., & Datta, A. (2008). The Child Attachment Interview: A psychometric study of reliability and discriminant validity. *Developmental Psychology, 44*, 939–956. http://dx.doi.org/10.1037/0012-1649.44.4.939

Contact person: Yael Shmueli-Goetz (Yael.Shmueli-Goetz@annafreud.org)

6. ASSESSMENT OF PLAY

Manual

Kernberg, O. F., & Normandin, L. (2000). *Children Play Therapy Instrument adapted for sexually abused children*. Unpublished manuscript, Cornell Medical School, New York Presbyterian Hospital, New York, NY.

Validation Articles

Kernberg, O. F., Chazan, S. E., & Normandin, L. (1998). The Children's Play Therapy Instrument (CPTI). *Journal of Psychotherapy Practice and Research, 7,* 196–207.

Tessier, V. P., Normandin, L., Ensink, K., & Fonagy, P. (2016). Fact or fiction? A longitudinal study of play and the development of reflective functioning. *Bulletin of the Menninger Clinic, 80,* 60–79. http://dx.doi.org/10.1521/bumc.2016.80.1.60

For a broader review of a range of measures to assess different elements of child and parental mentalizing or reflective functioning, see Vrouva, Target, and Ensink (2012).

REFERENCES

Abbass, A. A., Rabung, S., Leichsenring, F., Refseth, J. S., & Midgley, N. (2013). Psychodynamic psychotherapy for children and adolescents: A meta-analysis of short-term psychodynamic models. *Journal of the American Academy of Child & Adolescent Psychiatry, 52*, 863–875. http://dx.doi.org/10.1016/j.jaac.2013.05.014

Ainsworth, M. D. S., Blehar, M., Waters, E., & Wall, S. (1978). *Patterns of attachment: A psychological study of the Strange Situation.* Hillsdale, NJ: Erlbaum.

Allen, J. G. (2008). *Coping with trauma: Hope through understanding.* Arlington, VA: American Psychiatric Publishing.

Allen, J. G., & Fonagy, P. (Eds.). (2006). *The handbook of mentalization-based treatment.* http://dx.doi.org/10.1002/9780470712986

Allen, J. G., Fonagy, P., & Bateman, A. W. (2008). *Mentalizing in clinical practice.* Arlington, VA: American Psychiatric Publishing.

Allen, J. G., Lemma, A., & Fonagy, P. (2012). Trauma. In A. W. Bateman & P. Fonagy (Eds.), *Handbook of mentalizing in mental health practice* (pp. 419–444). Arlington, VA: American Psychiatric Publishing.

Allen, J. G., O'Malley, F., Freeman, C., & Bateman, A. W. (2012). Brief treatment. In A. W. Bateman & P. Fonagy (Eds.), *Handbook of mentalizing in mental health practice* (pp. 159–197). Arlington, VA: American Psychiatric Publishing.

Aron, E. N., Aron, A., & Davies, K. M. (2005). Adult shyness: The interaction of temperamental sensitivity and an adverse childhood environment. *Personality and Social Psychology Bulletin, 31*, 181–197. http://dx.doi.org/10.1177/0146167204271419

Asen, E., Bevington, D., Brasnett, H., Fearon, P., Fonagy, P., Keaveny, E., . . . Wood, S. (2011). *Mentalization-based treatment for families (MBT–F): Training slides.* Unpublished manuscript, Anna Freud Centre/University College London, London, England.

Asen, E., & Fonagy, P. (2012a). Mentalization-based family therapy. In A. W. Bateman & P. Fonagy (Eds.), *Handbook of mentalizing in mental health practice* (pp. 107–129). Arlington, VA: American Psychiatric Publishing.

Asen, E., & Fonagy, P. (2012b). Mentalization-based therapeutic interventions for families. *Journal of Family Therapy, 34*, 347–370. http://dx.doi.org/10.1111/j.1467-6427.2011.00552.x

Bak, P. L. (2012). "Thoughts in mind": Promoting mentalizing communities for children. In N. Midgley & I. Vrouva (Eds.), *Minding the child: Mentalization-based interventions with children and families* (pp. 202–218). London, England: Routledge.

Bak, P. L., Midgley, N., Zhu, J. L., Wistoft, K., & Obel, C. (2015). The Resilience Program: Preliminary evaluation of a mentalization-based education program. *New Frontiers of Psychology, 6*, 753.

Bakermans-Kranenburg, M. J., van IJzendoorn, M. H., & Juffer, F. (2003). Less is more: Meta-analyses of sensitivity and attachment interventions in early childhood. *Psychological Bulletin, 129*, 195–215. http://dx.doi.org/10.1037/0033-2909.129.2.195

Bammens, A. S., Adkins, T., & Badger, J. (2015). Psycho-educational intervention increases reflective functioning in foster and adoptive parents. *Adoption & Fostering, 39*, 38–50. http://dx.doi.org/10.1177/0308575914565069

Banerjee, R. (2008). Social cognition and anxiety in children. In C. Sharp, P. Fonagy, & I. Goodyer (Eds.), *Social cognition and developmental psychopathology* (pp. 239–270). http://dx.doi.org/10.1093/med/9780198569183.003.0009

Barish, K. (2009). *Emotions in child therapy.* New York, NY: Oxford University Press.

Baron-Cohen, S. (2009). Autism: The empathizing–systemizing (E-S) theory. *Annals of the New York Academy of Sciences, 1156*, 68–80. http://dx.doi.org/10.1111/j.1749-6632.2009.04467.x

Baron-Cohen, S., Leslie, A. M., & Frith, U. (1985). Does the autistic child have a "theory of mind"? *Cognition, 21*, 37–46.

Bateman, A. W., & Fonagy, P. (2004). Mentalization based treatment of BPD. *Journal of Personality Disorders, 18*, 36–51. http://dx.doi.org/10.1521/pedi.18.1.36.32772

Bateman, A. W., & Fonagy, P. (2006). *Mentalization-based treatment for borderline personality disorder: A practical guide.* http://dx.doi.org/10.1093/med/9780198570905.001.0001

Bateman, A. W., & Fonagy, P. (2009). Randomized controlled trial of outpatient mentalization-based treatment versus structured clinical management for borderline personality disorder. *The American Journal of Psychiatry, 166*, 1355–1364. Retrieved from http://ajp.psychiatryonline.org/doi/full/10.1176/appi.ajp.2009.09040539

Bateman, A. W., & Fonagy, P. (2010). Mentalization based treatment for borderline personality disorder. *World Psychiatry, 9*, 11–15. http://dx.doi.org/10.1002/j.2051-5545.2010.tb00255.x

Bateman, A. W., & Fonagy, P. (2012). Individual techniques of the basic model. In A. W. Bateman & P. Fonagy (Eds.), *Handbook of mentalizing in mental health practice* (pp. 67–80). Arlington, VA: American Psychiatric Publishing.

Bateman, A. W., & Fonagy, P. (2013). Mentalization-based treatment. *Psychoanalytic Inquiry, 33*, 595–613. http://dx.doi.org/10.1080/07351690.2013.835170

Bateman, A. W., & Fonagy, P. (2016). *Mentalization-based treatment for personality disorders: A practical guide.* Oxford, England: Oxford University Press.

Baumrind, D. (1966). Effects of authoritative parental control on child behavior. *Child Development, 37*, 887–907.

Beebe, B., Lachmann, F., & Jaffe, J. (1997). Mother–infant interaction structures and presymbolic self- and object representations. *Psychoanalytic Dialogues, 7*, 133–182. http://dx.doi.org/10.1080/10481889709539172

Beebe, B., Lachmann, F., Markese, S., Buck, K. A., Bahrick, L. E., Chen, H., . . . Jaffe, J. (2012). On the origins of disorganized attachment and internal working models: Paper II. An empirical microanalysis of 4-month mother–infant interaction. *Psychoanalytic Dialogues, 22*, 352–374. http://dx.doi.org/10.1080/10481885.2012.679606

Beebe, B., & Stern, D. (1977). Engagement-disengagement and early object experiences. In N. Freedman & S. Grand (Eds.), *Communicative structures and psychic structures* (pp. 35–55). http://dx.doi.org/10.1007/978-1-4757-0492-1_3

Benbassat, N., & Priel, B. (2012). Parenting and adolescent adjustment: The role of parental reflective functioning. *Journal of Adolescence, 35*, 163–174. http://dx.doi.org/10.1016/j.adolescence.2011.03.004

Berk, L. E., Mann, T. D., & Ogan, A. T. (2006). Make-believe play: Wellspring for the development of self-regulation. In D. G. Singer, R. Golinkoff, & K. Hirsh-Pasek (Eds.), *Play = learning: How play motivates and enhances children's cognitive and social-emotional growth* (pp. 74–100). http://dx.doi.org/10.1093/acprof:oso/9780195304381.003.0005

Berthelot, N., Ensink, K., Bernazzani, O., Normandin, L., Luyten, P., & Fonagy, P. (2015). Intergenerational transmission of attachment in abused and neglected mothers: The role of trauma-specific reflective functioning. *Infant Mental Health Journal, 36*, 200–212. http://dx.doi.org/10.1002/imhj.21499

Berthelot, N., Paccalet, T., Gilbert, E., Moreau, I., Mérette, C., Gingras, N., . . . Maziade, M. (2015). Childhood abuse and neglect may induce deficits in cognitive precursors of psychosis in high-risk children. *Journal of Psychiatry and Neuroscience, 40*, 336–343. http://dx.doi.org/10.1503/jpn.140211

Bevington, D. (Ed.). (n.d.). *MBT–F Core: Mentalization-based treatment for families*. Retrieved from http://mbtf.tiddlyspace.com/#

Bevington, D., & Fuggle, P. W. (2012). Supporting and enhancing mentalization in community outreach teams working with "hard to reach" youth: the AMBIT approach. In N. Midgley & J. Vrouva (Eds.), *Minding the child: Mentalization-based interventions with children, young people and their families* (pp. 163–186). London, England: Routledge.

Bevington, D., Fuggle, P., & Fonagy, P. (2015). Applying attachment theory to effective practice with hard-to-reach youth: The AMBIT approach. *Attachment & Human Development, 17*, 157–174. http://dx.doi.org/10.1080/14616734.2015.1006385

Bifulco, A., Moran, P. M., Ball, C., & Bernazzani, O. (2002). Adult attachment style: I. Its relationship to clinical depression. *Social Psychiatry and Psychiatric Epidemiology, 37*, 50–59. http://dx.doi.org/10.1007/s127-002-8215-0

Blake, P. (2008). *Child and adolescent psychotherapy*. London, England: Karnac Books.

Bleiberg, E. (2013). Mentalizing-based treatment with adolescents and families. *Child and Adolescent Psychiatric Clinics of North America, 22*, 295–330. http://dx.doi.org/10.1016/j.chc.2013.01.001

Bukatko, D., & Daehler, M. W. (2004). *Child development: A thematic approach* (5th ed.). Boston, MA: Houghton Mifflin.

Bunday, L., Dallos, R., Morgan, K., & McKenzie, R. (2015). Foster carers' reflective understandings of parenting looked after children: An exploratory study. *Adoption & Fostering*, *39*, 145–158. http://dx.doi.org/10.1177/0308575915588730

Capobianco, J., & Farber, B. A. (2005). Therapist self-disclosure to child patients. *American Journal of Psychotherapy*, *59*, 199–212.

Caspi, A., Houts, R. M., Belsky, D. W., Goodman-Mellor, S. J., Harrington, H., Israel, S., . . . Moffitt, T. E. (2014). The p factor: One general psychopathology factor in the structure of psychiatric disorders? *Clinical Psychological Science*, *2*, 119–137.

Cassidy, K. W., Werner, R. S., Rourke, M., Zubernis, L. S., & Balaraman, G. (2003). The relationship between psychological understanding and positive social behaviors. *Social Development*, *12*, 198–221. http://dx.doi.org/10.1111/1467-9507.00229

Centifanti, L. C., Meins, E., & Fernyhough, C. (2016). Callous-unemotional traits and impulsivity: Distinct longitudinal relations with mind-mindedness and understanding of others. *Journal of Child Psychology and Psychiatry*, *57*, 84–92. http://dx.doi.org/10.1111/jcpp.12445

Chazan, S., Kuchirko, Y., Beebe, B., & Sossin, K. M. (2016). A longitudinal study of traumatic play activity using the Children's Developmental Play Instrument (CDPI). *Journal of Infant, Child, & Adolescent Psychotherapy*, *15*, 1–25. http://dx.doi.org/10.1080/15289168.2015.1127729

Choi-Kain, L. W., & Gunderson, J. G. (2008). Mentalization: Ontogeny, assessment, and application in the treatment of borderline personality disorder. *The American Journal of Psychiatry*, *165*, 1127–1135. http://dx.doi.org/10.1176/appi.ajp.2008.07081360

Cicchetti, D., & Banny, A. (2014). A developmental psychopathology perspective on child maltreatment. In M. Lewis & K. D. Rudolph (Eds.), *Handbook of developmental psychopathology* (pp. 723–741). http://dx.doi.org/10.1007/978-1-4614-9608-3_37

Cicchetti, D., & Rogosch, F. A. (1996). Equifinality and multifinality in developmental psychopathology. *Development and Psychopathology*, *8*, 597–600. http://dx.doi.org/10.1017/S0954579400007318

Cicchetti, D., Rogosch, F. A., Maughan, A., Toth, S. L., & Bruce, J. (2003). False belief understanding in maltreated children. *Development and Psychopathology*, *15*, 1067–1091. http://dx.doi.org/10.1017/S0954579403000440

Clarke-Stewart, A., & Dunn, J. (Eds.). (2006). *Families count: Effects on child and adolescent development*. http://dx.doi.org/10.1017/CBO9780511616259

Cooper, A., & Redfern, S. (2016). *Reflective parenting: A guide to understanding what's going on in your child's mind*. New York, NY: Routledge.

Csibra, G., & Gergely, G. (2009). Natural pedagogy. *Trends in Cognitive Sciences*, *13*, 148–153. http://dx.doi.org/10.1016/j.tics.2009.01.005

Denham, S. A., Bassett, H. H., Way, E., Kalb, S., Warren-Khot, H., & Zinsser, K. (2014). "How would you feel? What would you do?" Development and underpinnings of preschoolers' social information processing. *Journal of Research in Childhood Education*, 28, 182–202. http://dx.doi.org/10.1080/02568543.2014.883558

Denham, S. A., & Kochanoff, A. T. (2002a). Parental contributions to preschoolers' understanding of emotion. *Marriage & Family Review*, 34, 311–343. http://dx.doi.org/10.1300/J002v34n03_06

Denham, S. A., & Kochanoff, A. T. (2002b). "Why is she crying?" Children's understanding of emotion from preschool to preadolescence. In L. F. Barrett & P. Salovey (Eds.), *The wisdom in feeling: Psychological processes in emotional intelligence* (pp. 239–270). New York, NY: Guilford Press.

Dodge, K. A., Laird, R., Lochman, J. E., Zelli, A., & the Conduct Problems Prevention Research Group. (2002). Multidimensional latent-construct analysis of children's social information processing patterns: Correlations with aggressive behavior problems. *Psychological Assessment*, 14, 60–73. http://dx.doi.org/10.1037/1040-3590.14.1.60

Dorahy, M. J., Middleton, W., Seager, L., Williams, M., & Chambers, R. (2016). Child abuse and neglect in complex dissociative disorder, abuse-related chronic PTSD, and mixed psychiatric samples. *Journal of Trauma & Dissociation*, 17, 223–236. http://dx.doi.org/10.1080/15299732.2015.1077916

Dunn, J., & Brown, J. (1994). Affect expression in the family, children's understanding of emotions, and their interactions with others. *Merrill-Palmer Quarterly*, 40, 120–137.

Dunn, J., Slomkowski, C., Donelan, N., & Herrera, C. (1995). Conflict, understanding, and relationships: developments and differences in the preschool years. *Early Education and Development*, 6, 303–316. http://dx.doi.org/10.1207/s15566935eed0604_2

Dvir, Y., Ford, J. D., Hill, M., & Frazier, J. A. (2014). Childhood maltreatment, emotional dysregulation, and psychiatric comorbidities. *Harvard Review of Psychiatry*, 22, 149–161. http://dx.doi.org/10.1097/HRP.0000000000000014

Eggum, N. D., Eisenberg, N., Kao, K., Spinrad, T. L., Bolnick, R., Hofer, C., . . . Fabricius, W. V. (2011). Emotion understanding, theory of mind, and prosocial orientation: Relations over time in early childhood. *The Journal of Positive Psychology*, 6, 4–16. http://dx.doi.org/10.1080/17439760.2010.536776

Emanuel, L. (2002). Deprivation × three: The contribution of organisational dynamics to the "triple deprivation" of looked after children. *Journal of Child Psychotherapy*, 28, 163–179. http://dx.doi.org/10.1080/00754170210143771

Ensink, K., Bégin, M., Normandin, L., Biberdzic, M., Vohl, G., & Fonagy, P. (2016). Le fonctionnement réflexif maternel et les symptômes intériorisés et extériorisés d'enfants victimes d'une agression sexuelle [Maternal reflective functioning and child internalizing and externalizing difficulties in the context of child sexual abuse]. *Revue Québécoise de Psychologie*, 37(3), 117–133.

Ensink, K., Bégin, M., Normandin, L., & Fonagy, P. (2016). Maternal and child reflective functioning in the context of child sexual abuse: Pathways to depression and externalising difficulties. *European Journal of Psychotraumatology*, 7, 30611. http://dx.doi.org/10.3402/ejpt.v7.30611

Ensink, K., Bégin, M., Normandin, L., Godbout, N., & Fonagy, P. (2016). Mentalization and dissociation in the context of trauma: Implications for child psychopathology. *Journal of Trauma & Dissociation*, 1–20. Advance online publication. http://dx.doi.org/10.1080/15299732.2016.1172536

Ensink, K., Berthelot, N., Bernazzani, O., Normandin, L., & Fonagy, P. (2014). Another step closer to measuring the ghosts in the nursery: Preliminary validation of the Trauma Reflective Functioning Scale. *Frontiers in Psychology*, 5, 1471. http://dx.doi.org/10.3389/fpsyg.2014.01471

Ensink, K., Berthelot, N., Biberdzic, M., & Normandin, L. (2016). The mirror paradigm: Assessing the embodied self in the context of abuse. *Psychoanalytic Psychology*, 33, 389–405. Advance online publication. http://dx.doi.org/10.1037/pap0000018

Ensink, K., Leroux, A., Normandin, L., Biberdzic, M., & Fonagy, P. (in press). Assessing reflective parenting in interaction with school-aged children. *Journal of Personality Assessment*.

Ensink, K., & Mayes, L. C. (2010). The development of mentalization in children from a theory of mind perspective. *Psychoanalytic Inquiry*, 30, 301–337. http://dx.doi.org/10.1080/07351690903206504

Ensink, K., & Normandin, L. (2011). Le traitement basé sur la mentalization chez des enfants agressés sexuellement et leurs parents [Mentalization therapy for sexually abused children and their parents]. In M. Hébert, M. Cyr, & M. Tourigny (Eds.), *L'agression sexuelle envers les enfants* [Sexual aggression toward children] (pp. 399–444). Collection Santé et Société. Montréal, Canada: Presse de l'Université du Québec.

Ensink, K., Normandin, L., Plamondon, A., Berthelot, N., & Fonagy, P. (2016). Intergenerational pathways from reflective functioning to infant attachment through parenting. *Canadian Journal of Behavioral Science/Revue Canadienne des sciences du comportement*, 48, 9.

Ensink, K., Normandin, L., Target, M., Fonagy, P., Sabourin, S., & Berthelot, N. (2015). Mentalization in children and mothers in the context of trauma: An initial study of the validity of the Child Reflective Functioning Scale. *British Journal of Developmental Psychology*, 33, 203–217. http://dx.doi.org/10.1111/bjdp.12074

Ensink, K., Target, M., Oandasan, C., & Duval, J. (2015). *Child Reflective Functioning Scale scoring manual: For application to the child attachment interview.* Unpublished manuscript, Anna Freud Centre/University College London, London, England.

Etezady, M. H., & Davis, M. (Eds.). (2012). *Clinical perspectives on reflective parenting: Keeping the child's mind in mind.* Plymouth, England: Aronson.

Fearon, P., & Belsky, J. (2004). Attachment and attention: Protection in relation to gender and cumulative social-contextual adversity. *Child Development*, 75, 1677–1693.

Fearon, P., Target, M., Sargent, J., Williams, L. L., McGregor, J., Bleiberg, E., & Fonagy, P. (2006). Short-term mentalization and relational therapy (SMART): An integrative family therapy for children and adolescents. In J. G. Allen & P. Fonagy (Eds.), *Handbook of mentalization-based treatment* (pp. 201–222). Chichester, England: John Wiley & Sons.

Fischer-Kern, M., Fonagy, P., Kapusta, N. D., Luyten, P., Boss, S., Naderer, A., . . . Leithner, K. (2013). Mentalizing in female inpatients with major depressive disorder. *Journal of Nervous and Mental Disease, 201*, 202–207. http://dx.doi.org/10.1097/NMD.0b013e3182845c0a

Fonagy, P. (1991). Thinking about thinking: Some clinical and theoretical considerations in the treatment of a borderline patient. *The International Journal of Psychoanalysis, 72*, 639–656.

Fonagy, P. (2004). Early-life trauma and the psychogenesis and prevention of violence. *Annals of the New York Academy of Sciences, 1036*, 181–200. http://dx.doi.org/10.1196/annals.1330.012

Fonagy, P. (2015). Mutual regulation, mentalization and therapeutic action: A reflection on the contributions of Ed Tronick to developmental and psychotherapeutic thinking. *Psychoanalytic Inquiry, 35*, 355–369. http://dx.doi.org/10.1080/07351690.2015.1022481

Fonagy, P., & Allison, E. (2012). What is mentalization? The concept and its foundations in developmental research. In N. Midgley & I. Vrouva (Eds.), *Minding the child: Mentalization-based interventions with children, young people and their families* (pp. 11–34). London, England: Routledge.

Fonagy, P., & Allison, E. (2014). The role of mentalizing and epistemic trust in the therapeutic relationship. *Psychotherapy, 51*, 372–380. http://dx.doi.org/10.1037/a0036505

Fonagy, P., & Bateman, A. W. (2006). Mechanisms of change in mentalization-based treatment of BPD. *Journal of Clinical Psychology, 62*, 411–430. http://dx.doi.org/10.1002/jclp.20241

Fonagy, P., & Bateman, A. W. (2007). Mentalizing and borderline personality disorder. *Journal of Mental Health, 16*, 83–101. http://dx.doi.org/10.1080/09638230601182045

Fonagy, P., & Campbell, C. (2015). Bad blood revisited: Attachment and psychoanalysis, 2015. *British Journal of Psychotherapy, 31*, 229–250. http://dx.doi.org/10.1111/bjp.12150

Fonagy, P., Gergely, G., Jurist, E., & Target, M. (2002). *Affect regulation, mentalization and the development of the self*. New York, NY: Other Press.

Fonagy, P., Gergely, G., & Target, M. (2007). The parent–infant dyad and the construction of the subjective self. *Journal of Child Psychology and Psychiatry, 48*, 288–328. http://dx.doi.org/10.1111/j.1469-7610.2007.01727.x

Fonagy, P., Luyten, P., & Allison, E. (2015). Epistemic petrification and the restoration of epistemic trust: A new conceptualization of borderline personality disorder and its psychosocial treatment. *Journal of Personality Disorders, 29*, 575–609. http://dx.doi.org/10.1521/pedi.2015.29.5.575

Fonagy, P., Luyten, P., Allison, E., & Campbell, C. (2016). Reconciling psychoanalytic ideas with attachment theory. In J. Cassidy & P. R. Shaver (Eds.), *Handbook of attachment* (3rd ed., pp. 780–804). New York, NY: Guilford Press.

Fonagy, P., Steele, M., Steele, H., Higgitt, A., & Target, M. (1994). The Emanuel Miller Memorial Lecture 1992: The theory and practice of resilience. *Journal of Child Psychology and Psychiatry, and Allied Disciplines, 35*, 231–257. Retrieved from http://www.ncbi.nlm.nih.gov/pubmed/8188797

Fonagy, P., Steele, M., Steele, H., Moran, G. S., & Higgitt, A. C. (1991). The capacity for understanding mental states: The reflective self in parent and child and its significance for security of attachment. *Infant Mental Health Journal, 12*, 201–218. http://dx.doi.org/10.1002/1097-0355(199123)12:3<201::AID-IMHJ2280120307>3.0.CO;2-7

Fonagy, P., & Target, M. (1996a). A contemporary psychoanalytic perspective: Psychodynamic developmental therapy. In E. Hibbs & P. Jensen (Eds.), *Psychosocial treatments for child and adolescent disorders: Empirically based strategies for clinical practice* (pp. 619–638). http://dx.doi.org/10.1037/10196-024

Fonagy, P., & Target, M. (1996b). Playing with reality: I. Theory of mind and the normal development of psychic reality. *The International Journal of Psychoanalysis, 77*, 217–233.

Fonagy, P., & Target, M. (1997). Attachment and reflective function: Their role in self-organization. *Development and Psychopathology, 9*, 679–700. http://dx.doi.org/10.1017/S0954579497001399

Fonagy, P., & Target, M. (1998). Mentalization and the changing aims of child psychoanalysis. *Psychoanalytic Dialogues, 8*, 87–114. http://dx.doi.org/10.1080/10481889809539235

Fonagy, P., & Target, M. (2000). Playing with reality: III. The persistence of dual psychic reality in borderline patients. *The International Journal of Psychoanalysis, 81*, 853–873.

Fonagy, P., & Target, M. (2002). Early intervention and the development of self-regulation. *Psychoanalytic Inquiry, 22*, 307–335. http://dx.doi.org/10.1080/07351692209348990

Fonagy, P., & Target, M. (2006). The mentalization-focused approach to self pathology. *Journal of Personality Disorders, 20*, 544–576. http://dx.doi.org/10.1521/pedi.2006.20.6.544

Fonagy, P., & Target, M. (2007a). Playing with reality: IV. A theory of external reality rooted in intersubjectivity. *The International Journal of Psychoanalysis, 88*, 917–937. http://dx.doi.org/10.1516/4774-6173-241T-7225

Fonagy, P., & Target, M. (2007b). The rooting of the mind in the body: New links between attachment theory and psychoanalytic thought. *Journal of the American Psychoanalytic Association, 55*, 411–456. http://dx.doi.org/10.1177/00030651070550020501

Fragkiadaki, E., & Strauss, S. M. (2012). Termination of psychotherapy: The journey of 10 psychoanalytic and psychodynamic therapists. *Psychology and Psycho-*

therapy: Theory, Research and Practice, 85, 335–350. http://dx.doi.org/10.1111/j.2044-8341.2011.02035.x

Fraiberg, S., Adelson, E., & Shapiro, V. (1975). Ghosts in the nursery: A psychoanalytic approach to the problems of impaired infant–mother relationships. Journal of the American Academy of Child Psychiatry, 14, 387–421. http://dx.doi.org/10.1016/S0002-7138(09)61442-4

Fredrickson, B. L. (2001). The role of positive emotions on positive psychology. The broaden-and-build theory of passive emotions. American Psychologist, 56, 218–226.

Freud, A. (1965). Normality and pathology in childhood: Assessments of development. London, England: Hogarth Press.

Freyd, J., & Birrell, P. (2013). Blind to betrayal: Why we fool ourselves we aren't being fooled. Hoboken, NJ: Wiley.

Frith, U. (2004). Emanuel Miller lecture: Confusions and controversies about Asperger syndrome. Journal of Child Psychology and Psychiatry, 45, 672–686. http://dx.doi.org/10.1111/j.1469-7610.2004.00262.x

Fuggle, P., Bevington, D., Cracknell, L., Hanley, J., Hare, S., Lincoln, J., . . . Zlotowitz, S. (2015). The adolescent mentalization-based integrative treatment (AMBIT) approach to outcome evaluation and manualization: Adopting a learning organization approach. Clinical Child Psychology and Psychiatry, 20, 419–435. http://dx.doi.org/10.1177/1359104514521640

George, C., Kaplan, N., & Main, M. (1996). Adult Attachment Interview Protocol (3rd ed.). Unpublished manuscript, University of California at Berkeley.

Gergely, G., & Watson, J. S. (1996). The social biofeedback theory of parental affect-mirroring: The development of emotional self-awareness and self-control in infancy. The International Journal of Psychoanalysis, 77, 1181–1212.

Gergely, G., & Watson, J. S. (1999). Early socio-emotional development: Contingency perception and the social-biofeedback model. In P. Rochat (Ed.), Early social cognition: Understanding others in the first months of life (pp. 101–136). Mahwah, NJ: Erlbaum.

Gil, E., & Crenshaw, D. A. (2016). Termination challenges in child psychotherapy. New York, NY: Guilford Press.

Gil, E., & Drewes, A. A. (2005). Cultural issues in play therapy. New York, NY: Guilford Press.

Gluckers, G., & Van Lier, L. (2011). Beeld en betekenis. Sleutelscènes uit de opleiding tot kindertherapeut [Images and meaning: Decisive moments in the education of a child psychotherapist]. Tijdschrift voor Psychoanalyse, 17, 150–163.

Golding, K. S. (2015). Connection before correction: Supporting parents to meet the challenges of parenting children who have been traumatised within their early parenting environments. Children Australia, 40, 152–159. http://dx.doi.org/10.1017/cha.2015.9

Goodman, G., Midgley, N., & Schneider, C. (2016). Expert clinicians' prototypes of an ideal child treatment in psychodynamic and cognitive-behavioral therapy: Is mentalization seen as a common process factor? *Psychotherapy Research, 26,* 590–601. http://dx.doi.org/10.1080/10503307.2015.1049672

Goodman, G., Reed, P., & Athey-Lloyd, L. (2015). Mentalization and play therapy processes between two therapists and a child with Asperger's disorder. *International Journal of Play Therapy, 24,* 13–29. http://dx.doi.org/10.1037/a0038660

Goodman, G., Stroh, M., & Valdez, A. (2012). Do attachment representations predict depression and anxiety in psychiatrically hospitalized prepubertal children? *Bulletin of the Menninger Clinic, 76,* 260–289. http://dx.doi.org/10.1521/bumc.2012.76.3.260

Green, H., McGinnity, Á., Meltzer, H., Ford, T., & Goodman, R. (2005). *Mental health of children and young people in Great Britain, 2004.* Basingstoke, England: Palgrave Macmillan.

Greenspan, S. I. (1997). *Developmentally based psychotherapy.* Madison, CT: International Universities Press.

Gydal, M., & Knudtzon, S. (2002). Om tidsbegrenset psykoterapi med barn [On time-limited psychotherapy with children]. *Tidsskrift for Norsk Psykologforening, 39,* 911–915.

Hagell, A., & Maughan, B. (in press). Epidemiology: Are mental health problems in children and young people really a big issue? In N. Midgley, J. Hayes, & M. Cooper (Eds.), *Essential research findings in child and adolescent counselling and psychotherapy.* London, England: Sage.

Happé, F., & Frith, U. (2014). Annual research review: Towards a developmental neuroscience of atypical social cognition. *Journal of Child Psychology and Psychiatry, 55,* 553–577. http://dx.doi.org/10.1111/jcpp.12162

Harter, S. (2012). *The construction of the self: Developmental and sociocultural foundations* (2nd ed.). New York, NY: Guilford Press.

Haslam-Hopwood, G. T. G., Allen, J. G., Stein, A., & Bleiberg, E. (2006). Enhancing mentalizing through psycho-education. In J. G. Allen & P. Fonagy (Eds.), *Handbook of mentalization-based treatment* (pp. 249–267). http://dx.doi.org/10.1002/9780470712986.ch13

Haugvik, M. (2013). Structured parallel therapy with parents in time-limited psychotherapy with children experiencing difficult family situations. *Clinical Child Psychology and Psychiatry, 18,* 504–518. http://dx.doi.org/10.1177/1359104512460859

Haugvik, M., & Johns, U. (2006). Betydningen av felles fokus i tidsavgrenset psykoterapi med barn: En kvalitativ studie av psykoterapi med barn som opplever vanskelige familieforhold [The significance of a shared focus in time-limited psychotherapy with children: A qualitative study of psychotherapy with children experiencing difficult family circumstances]. *Tidsskrift for Norsk Psykologforening, 43,* 19–29.

Haugvik, M., & Johns, U. (2008). Facets of structure and adaptation: A qualitative study of time-limited psychotherapy with children experiencing difficult family situations. *Clinical Child Psychology and Psychiatry*, *13*, 235–252. http://dx.doi.org/10.1177/1359104507088345

Hertzmann, L., & Abse, S. (2010). *Mentalization based treatment for inter-parental conflict (Parenting Together): A treatment manual.* Unpublished manuscript, The Tavistock Centre for Couple Relationships, London, England.

Hodges, J., Steele, M., Hillman, S., Henderson, K., & Kaniuk, J. (2003). Changes in attachment representations over the first year of adoptive placement: Narratives of maltreated children. *Clinical Child Psychology and Psychiatry*, *8*, 351–367. http://dx.doi.org/10.1177/1359104503008003006

Hoffman, L., Rice, T., & Prout, T. (2016). *Manual of regulation-focused psychotherapy for children (RFP-C) with externalizing behaviors: A psychodynamic approach.* London, England: Routledge.

Hughes, C., & Ensor, R. (2008). Social cognition and disruptive behavior disorder in young children: Families matter. In C. Sharp, P. Fonagy, & I. Goodyer (Eds.), *Social cognition and developmental psychopathology* (pp. 115–140). http://dx.doi.org/10.1093/med/9780198569183.003.0005

Hughes, D. A. (2000). *Facilitating developmental attachment: The road to emotional recovery and behavioral change in foster and adopted children.* Oxford, England: Aronson.

Hughes, D. A. (2004). An attachment-based treatment of maltreated children and young people. *Attachment & Human Development*, *6*, 263–278. http://dx.doi.org/10.1080/14616730412331281539

Hurry, A. (Ed.). (1998). *Psychoanalysis and developmental therapy* [Psychoanalytic Monograph No. 3]. London, England: Karnac Books.

Jacob, J., Edbrooke-Childs, J., Law, D., & Wolpert, M. (2015). Measuring what matters to patients: Using goal content to inform measure choice and development. *Clinical Child Psychology and Psychiatry*. Advance online publication. http://dx.doi.org/10.1177/1359104515615642

Jacobsen, M. N., Ha, C., & Sharp, C. (2015). A mentalization-based treatment approach to caring for youth in foster care. *Journal of Infant, Child, and Adolescent Psychotherapy*, *14*, 440–454. http://dx.doi.org/10.1080/15289168.2015.1093921

Johns, U. (2008). "Å bruke tiden—hva betyr egentlig det?" Tid og relasjon—et intersubjektivt perspektiv ["To make use of time—what does that really mean?" Time and relationships—an intersubjective perspective]. In G. Trondalen & E. Ruud (Eds.), *Perspektiver på musikk og helse: Skriftserie fra Senter for musikk og helse* (pp. 67–83). Oslo, Norway: NMH.

Johnson, D. E. (2000). Medical and developmental sequelae of early childhood institutionalization in international adoptees from Romania and the Russian Federation. In C. A. Nelson (Ed.), *The effects of adversity on neurobehavioral development* (pp. 113–162). Mahwah, NJ: Erlbaum.

Johnson, D. E. (2002). Adoption and the effect on children's development. *Early Human Development, 68,* 39–54. http://dx.doi.org/10.1016/S0378-3782(02)00017-8

Jurist, E. L. (2005). Mentalized affectivity. *Psychoanalytic Psychology, 22,* 426–444. http://dx.doi.org/10.1037/0736-9735.22.3.426

Keaveny, E., Midgley, N., Asen, E., Bevington, D., Fearon, P., Fonagy, P., . . . Wood, S. (2012). Minding the family mind: The development and initial evaluation of mentalization based treatment for families. In N. Midgley & I. Vrouva (Eds.), *Minding the child: Mentalization-based interventions with children, young people and their families* (pp. 98–112). London, England: Routledge.

Kegerreis, S., & Midgley, N. (2014). Psychodynamic approaches. In S. Pattison, M. Robson, & A. Beynon (Eds.), *The handbook of counselling children and young people* (pp. 35–48). London, England: Sage.

Kernberg, P. F., & Chazan, S. E. (1991). *Children with conduct disorders: A psychotherapy manual.* New York, NY: Basic Books.

Kernberg, P. F., Chazan, S. E., & Normandin, L. (1998). The Children's Play Therapy Instrument (CPTI): Description, development, and reliability studies. *Journal of Psychotherapy Practice and Research, 7,* 196–207.

Kernberg, P. F., Weiner, A. S., & Bardenstein, K. (2000). *Personality disorders in children and adolescents.* New York, NY: Basic Books.

Kim, S. (2015). The mind in the making: Developmental and neurobiological origins of mentalizing. *Personality Disorders: Theory, Research, and Practice, 6,* 356–365. http://dx.doi.org/10.1037/per0000102

Klimes-Dougan, B., & Kistner, J. (1990). Physically abused preschoolers' responses to peers' distress. *Developmental Psychology, 26,* 599–602. http://dx.doi.org/10.1037/0012-1649.26.4.599

Kochanska, G., Aksan, N., & Joy, M. E. (2007). Children's fearfulness as a moderator of parenting in early socialization: Two longitudinal studies. *Developmental Psychology, 43,* 222–237. http://dx.doi.org/10.1037/0012-1649.43.1.222

Kochanska, G., Coy, K. C., & Murray, K. T. (2001). The development of self-regulation in the first four years of life. *Child Development, 72,* 1091–1111. http://dx.doi.org/10.1111/1467-8624.00336

Koren-Karie, N., Oppenheim, D., Dolev, S., Sher, E., & Etzion-Carasso, A. (2002). Mothers' insightfulness regarding their infants' internal experience: Relations with maternal sensitivity and infant attachment. *Developmental Psychology, 38,* 534–542. http://dx.doi.org/10.1037/0012-1649.38.4.534

Kovács, Á. M., Téglás, E., & Endress, A. D. (2010). The social sense: Susceptibility to others' beliefs in human infants and adults. *Science, 330,* 1830–1834. http://dx.doi.org/10.1126/science.1190792

Kring, A. M. (2008). Emotion disturbances as transdiagnostic processes in psychopathology. In I. M. Lewis, J. M. Haviland-Jones, & L. F. Barrett (Eds.), *Handbook of emotions* (Vol. 3, pp. 691–705). New York, NY: Guilford Press.

Lanyado, M. (2012). Transition and change: An exploration of the resonance between transitional and meditative states of mind and their roles in the therapeutic process. In A. Horne & M. Lanyado (Eds.), *Winnicott's children: Independent psychoanalytic approaches with children and adolescents* (pp. 123–139). Hove, England; New York, NY: Routledge.

Laurent, G., & Ensink, K. (2016). *Emotional understanding, social adaptation, and aggression in 4-year-olds.* Manuscript submitted for publication.

Law, D., & Wolpert, M. (Eds.). (2014). *Guide to using outcomes and feedback tools with children, young people and families* (2nd ed.). London, England: CAMHS Press.

Lengua, L. J. (2008). Anxiousness, frustration, and effortful control as moderators of the relation between parenting and adjustment in middle-childhood. *Social Development, 17,* 554–577. http://dx.doi.org/10.1111/j.1467-9507.2007.00438.x

Liao, Z., Li, Y., & Su, Y. (2014). Emotion understanding and reconciliation in overt and relational conflict scenarios among preschoolers. *International Journal of Behavioral Development, 38,* 111–117. http://dx.doi.org/10.1177/0165025413512064

Lieberman, A., Padrón, E., Van Horn, P., & Harris, W. W. (2005). Angels in the nursery: The intergenerational transmission of benevolent parental influences. *Infant Mental Health Journal, 26,* 504–520. http://dx.doi.org/10.1002/imhj.20071

Lillard, A. S., Lerner, M. D., Hopkins, E. J., Dore, R. A., Smith, E. D., & Palmquist, C. M. (2013). The impact of pretend play on children's development: A review of the evidence. *Psychological Bulletin, 139,* 1–34. http://dx.doi.org/10.1037/a0029321

Luyten, P., & Fonagy, P. (2015). The neurobiology of mentalizing. *Personality Disorders: Theory, Research, and Treatment, 6,* 366–379. http://dx.doi.org/10.1037/per0000117

Luyten, P., Fonagy, P., Lemma, A., & Target, M. (2012). Depression. In A. W. Bateman & P. Fonagy (Eds.), *The handbook of mentalizing in mental health practice* (pp. 386–418). Arlington, VA: American Psychiatric Publishing.

Luyten, P., Fonagy, P., Lowyck, B., & Vermote, R. (2012). Assessment of mentalization. In A. W. Bateman & P. Fonagy (Eds.), *Handbook of mentalizing in mental health practice* (pp. 43–67). Arlington, VA: American Psychiatric Publishing.

Lyons-Ruth, K., Bruschweiler-Stern, N., Harrison, A. M., Morgan, A. C., Nahum, J. P., Sander, L., . . . Tronick, E. Z. (1998). Implicit relational knowing: Its role in development and psychoanalytic treatment. *Infant Mental Health, 19,* 281–289. http://dx.doi.org/10.1002/(SICI)1097-0355(199823)19:3<282::AID-IMHJ3>3.0.CO;2-O

Macfie, J., Cicchetti, D., & Toth, S. L. (2001). Dissociation in maltreated versus nonmaltreated preschool-aged children. *Child Abuse & Neglect, 25,* 1253–1267. http://dx.doi.org/10.1016/S0145-2134(01)00266-6

Malberg, N. T. (2015). Activating mentalization in parents: An integrative framework. *Journal of Infant, Child, and Adolescent Psychotherapy, 14,* 232–245. http://dx.doi.org/10.1080/15289168.2015.1068002

Malberg, N. T., & Fonagy, P. (2012). Creating security by exploring the personal meaning of chronic illness in adolescent patients. In M. O'Reilly-Landry (Ed.), *A psychodynamic understanding of modern medicine* (pp. 27–38). London, England: Radcliffe Press.

Marty, P. (1991). *Mentalization et psychosomatique* [Mentalization and psychosomatics]. Le Plessis-Robinson, France: Synthelabo, Collection Les Empêcheurs de Penser en Rond.

Mason, B. (1993). Towards positions of safe uncertainty. *Human Systems: The Journal of Systemic Consultation & Management, 4,* 189–200.

Masterpasqua, F. (2016). Mindfulness mentalizing humanism: A transtheoretical convergence. *Journal of Psychotherapy Integration, 26,* 5–10. http://dx.doi.org/10.1037/a0039635

McLaughlin, C., Holliday, C., Clarke, B., & Ilie, S. (2013). *Research on counselling and psychotherapy with children and young people: A systematic scoping review of the evidence for its effectiveness from 2003–2011.* Leicester, England: British Association for Counselling and Psychotherapy.

McMahon, L. (2009). *The handbook of play therapy and therapeutic play* (2nd ed.). Hove, England; New York, NY: Routledge.

Meins, E., Centifanti, L. C. M., Fernyhough, C., & Fishburn, S. (2013). Maternal mind-mindedness and children's behavioral difficulties: Mitigating the impact of low socioeconomic status. *Journal of Abnormal Child Psychology, 41,* 543–553. http://dx.doi.org/10.1007/s10802-012-9699-3

Meins, E., Fernyhough, C., Fradley, E., & Tuckey, M. (2001). Rethinking maternal sensitivity: Mothers' comments on infants' mental processes predict security of attachment at 12 months. *Journal of Child Psychology and Psychiatry, 42,* 637–648. http://dx.doi.org/10.1111/1469-7610.00759

Meins, E., Fernyhough, C., Wainwright, R., Clark-Carter, D., Das Gupta, M., Fradley, E., & Tuckey, M. (2003). Pathways to understanding mind: Construct validity and predictive validity of maternal mind-mindedness. *Child Development, 74,* 1194–1211. http://dx.doi.org/10.1111/1467-8624.00601

Midgley, N., Besser, S. J., Dye, H., Fearon, P., Gale, T., Jefferies-Sewell, K., . . . Wood, S. (2017). The Herts and Minds Study: Evaluating the effectiveness of mentalization-based treatment (MBT) as an intervention for children in foster care with emotional and/or behavioural problems: A Phase II, feasibility, randomised controlled trial. *Pilot and Feasibility Studies, 3,* 1–12. http://dx.doi.org/10.1186/s40814-017-0127-x

Midgley, N., & Vrouva, I. (Eds.). (2012). *Minding the child: Mentalization-based interventions with children, young people and their families.* London, England: Routledge.

Mikulincer, M., & Shaver, P. R. (2007). *Attachment in adulthood: Structure, dynamics, and change.* New York, NY: Guilford Press.

Moore, C., & Dunham, P. (1995). *Joint attention: Its origins and role in development.* Mahwah, NJ: Erlbaum.

Muller, N. (2009, November). *MBT in organizations: Improving the cooperation between a youth and adults department.* Lecture presented at the Conference of the Patient Association of Clients With Borderline Personality Disorder (Triade).

Muller, N. (2011). Mentaliseren bevorderende therapie voor families waarbij uithuisplaatsing dreigt of heeft plaats gevonden [Mentalization based treatment for families in which a child is placed in foster care or on the edge of care]. *Tijdschrift voor Kinder en Jeugdpsychotherapie, 38,* 47–57.

Muller, N., & Bakker, T. (2009). Oog voor de ouders: Diagnostiek van de hechtingsrelatie tussen ouders en kinderen en het mentaliserend vermogen van ouders [Eyes on the parent: Assessment of the attachment relationship between parents and their children and their mentalizing abilities]. *Tijdschrift voor Kinder en Jeugdpsychotherapie, 39,* 65–79.

Muller, N., Gerits, L., & Siecker, I. (2012). Mentalization-based therapies with adopted children and their families. In N. Midgley & I. Vrouva (Eds.), *Minding the child: Mentalization-based interventions with children, young people and their families* (pp. 113–130). London, England: Routledge.

Muller, N., & Midgley, N. (2015). Approaches to assessment in time-limited mentalization-based therapy for children (MBT–C). *Frontiers in Psychology, 6,* 1063.

Muller, N., & ten Kate, C. (2008). Mentaliseren bevorderende therapie in relaties en gezinnen [Mentalization based treatment in couples and family therapy]. *Tijdschrift voor Systeemtherapie, 20,* 117–132.

Muñoz Specht, P., Ensink, K., Normandin, L., & Midgley, N. (2016). Mentalizing techniques used by psychodynamic therapists working with children and early adolescents. *Bulletin of the Menninger Clinic, 80*(4), 281–315.

Murray, H. A. (1943). *Thematic Apperception Test: Manual.* Cambridge, MA: Harvard University Press.

Music, G. (2011). *Nurturing natures: Attachment and children's emotional, sociocultural and brain development.* New York, NY: Psychology Press.

Nelson, K. (2003). Narrative and self, myth and memory: Emergence of the cultural self. In R. Dans & C. A. Fivush (Eds.), *Autobiographical memory and the construction of a narrative self: Developmental and cultural perspectives* (pp. 3–28). Mahwah, NJ: Erlbaum.

Novick, K. K., & Novick, J. (2005). *Working with parents makes therapy work.* Plymouth, England: Rowman and Littlefield.

Nyberg, V., & Hertzmann, L. (2014). Developing a mentalization-based treatment (MBT) for therapeutic intervention with couples (MBT–CT). *Couple and Family Psychoanalysis, 4,* 116–135.

Ogrodniczuk, J. S., Joyce, A. S., & Piper, W. E. (2005). Strategies for reducing patient-initiated premature termination of psychotherapy. *Harvard Review of Psychiatry, 13,* 57–70. http://dx.doi.org/10.1080/10673220590956429

Ordway, M. R., Sadler, L. S., Dixon, J., Close, N., Mayes, L., & Slade, A. (2014). Lasting effects of an interdisciplinary home visiting program on child behavior: Preliminary follow-up results of a randomized trial. *Journal of Pediatric Nursing, 29*, 3–13. http://dx.doi.org/10.1016/j.pedn.2013.04.006

Ostler, T., Bahar, O. S., & Jessee, A. (2010). Mentalization in children exposed to parental methamphetamine abuse: Relations to children's mental health and behavioral outcomes. *Attachment & Human Development, 12*, 193–207. http://dx.doi.org/10.1080/14616731003759666

Pally, R., & Popek, P. (2012). CRP direct services and training programs. In M. H. Etezady & M. Davis (Eds.), *Clinical perspectives on reflective parenting: Keeping the child's mind in mind* (pp. 31–58). Plymouth, England: Aronson.

Panksepp, J. (2007). Can PLAY diminish ADHD and facilitate the construction of the social brain? *Journal of the Canadian Academy of Child and Adolescent Psychiatry, 16*, 57–66.

Panksepp, J., & Biven, L. (2012). *Archaeology of mind: The neuroevolutionary origins of human emotions.* New York, NY: Norton.

Pears, K. C., & Fisher, P. A. (2005). Emotion understanding and theory of mind among maltreated children in foster care: Evidence of deficits. *Development and Psychopathology, 17*, 47–65. http://dx.doi.org/10.1017/S0954579405050030

Perepletchikova, F., & Goodman, G. (2014). Two approaches to treating preadolescent children with severe emotional and behavioral problems: Dialectical behavior therapy adapted for children and mentalization-based child therapy. *Journal of Psychotherapy Integration, 24*, 298–312. http://dx.doi.org/10.1037/a0038134

Pons, F., Harris, P. L., & de Rosnay, M. (2004). Emotion comprehension between 3 and 11 years: Developmental periods and hierarchical organization. *European Journal of Developmental Psychology, 1*, 127–152. http://dx.doi.org/10.1080/17405620344000022

Premack, D., & Woodruff, G. (1978). Does the chimpanzee have a theory of mind? *Behavioral and Brain Sciences, 1*, 515–526. http://dx.doi.org/10.1017/S0140525X00076512

Putnam, F. W. (1997). *Dissociation in children and adolescents: A developmental perspective.* New York, NY: Guilford Press.

Ramchandani, P., & Jones, D. P. H. (2003). Treating psychological symptoms in sexually abused children: From research findings to service provision. *The British Journal of Psychiatry, 183*, 484–490.

Ramires, V. R. R., Schwan, S., & Midgley, N. (2012). Mentalization-based therapy with maltreated children living in shelters in southern Brazil: A single case study. *Psychoanalytic Psychotherapy, 26*, 308–326. http://dx.doi.org/10.1080/02668734.2012.730546

Rexwinkel, M. J., & Verheugt-Pleiter, A. J. E. (2008). Helping parents to promote mentalization. In A. J. E. Verheugt-Pleiter, J. Zevalkink, & M. G. J. Schmeets

(Eds.), *Mentalizing in child therapy: Guidelines for clinical practitioners* (pp. 69–90). London, England: Karnac Books.

Røed Hansen, B. (2012). *I dialog med barnet: Intersubjektivitet i utvikling og i psykoterapi* [In dialogue with the child: Intersubjectivity in development and in psychotherapy]. Oslo, Norway: Gyldendal.

Rogers, C. R. (1957). The necessary and sufficient conditions of therapeutic personality change. *Journal of Consulting Psychology, 21*, 95–103.

Rosenfeld, S. K., & Sprince, M. P. (1965). Some thoughts on the technical handling of borderline children. *The Psychoanalytic Study of the Child, 20*, 495–517.

Rosenstein, D. S., & Horowitz, H. A. (1996). Adolescent attachment and psychopathology. *Journal of Consulting and Clinical Psychology, 64*, 244–253. http://dx.doi.org/10.1037/0022-006X.64.2.244

Roskam, I., Stiévenart, M., Meunier, J. C., Van de Moortele, G., Kinoo, P., & Nassogne, M. C. (2011). Le diagnostic précoce des troubles du comportement externalisé est-il fiable? Mise à l'épreuve d'une procédure multi-informateurs et multiméthodes [Is the reliability of early diagnosis of externalizing behavior in question? Towards a multi-informant and multi-method strategy]. *Pratiques Psychologiques, 17*, 189–200. http://dx.doi.org/10.1016/j.prps.2009.07.001

Rossouw, T. (2012). Self-harm in young people. Is MBT the answer? In N. Midgley & I. Vrouva (Eds.), *Minding the child. Mentalization-based interventions with children, young people and their families* (pp. 131–144). London, England: Routledge.

Rossouw, T. I., & Fonagy, P. (2012). Mentalization-based treatment for self-harm in adolescents: A randomized controlled trial. *Journal of the American Academy of Child & Adolescent Psychiatry, 51*, 1304–1313.e3. http://dx.doi.org/10.1016/j.jaac.2012.09.018

Safran, J. D., & Muran, J. C. (2000). *Negotiating the therapeutic alliance: A relational treatment guide*. New York, NY: Guilford Press.

Safran, J. D., Muran, J. C., & Eubanks-Carter, C. (2011). Repairing alliance ruptures. *Psychotherapy, 48*, 80–87. http://dx.doi.org/10.1037/a0022140

Salyer, K. (2002, Autumn). Time-limited therapy: A necessary evil in the managed care era? *Reformulation*, 9–11.

Schaffer, H. R. (2006). *Key concepts in developmental psychology*. Thousand Oaks, CA: Sage.

Schore, A. N. (1994). *Affect regulation and the origin of the self*. Mahwah, NJ: Erlbaum.

Schore, A. N. (2003). *Affect regulation and the repair of the self*. New York, NY: Norton.

Scott, S., & Dadds, M. R. (2009). Practitioner review: When parent training doesn't work: Theory-driven clinical strategies. *Journal of Child Psychology and Psychiatry, and Allied Disciplines, 50*, 1441–1450. http://dx.doi.org/10.1111/j.1469-7610.2009.02161.x

Shai, D., & Fonagy, P. (2014). Beyond words: Parental embodied mentalizing and the parent–infant dance. In M. Mikulincer & P. R. Shaver (Eds.), *Mechanisms of social connection: From brain to group* (pp. 185–203). http://dx.doi.org/10.1037/14250-011

Sharp, C. (2006). Mentalizing problems in childhood disorders. In J. G. Allen & P. Fonagy (Eds.), *Handbook of mentalization-based treatments* (pp. 101–121). Chichester, England: Wiley.

Sharp, C., Fonagy, P., & Goodyer, I. (Eds.). (2008). *Social cognition and developmental psychopathology.* http://dx.doi.org/10.1093/med/9780198569183.001.0001

Sharp, C., Ha, C., & Fonagy, P. (2011). Get them before they get you: Trust, trustworthiness, and social cognition in boys with and without externalizing behavior problems. *Development and Psychopathology, 23,* 647–658. http://dx.doi.org/10.1017/S0954579410000003

Sharp, C., & Venta, A. (2012). Mentalizing problems in children and adolescents. In N. Midgley & I. Vrouva (Eds.), *Minding the child: Mentalization-based interventions with children, young people and their families* (pp. 35–53). London, England: Routledge.

Sharp, C., Williams, L. L., Ha, C., Baumgardner, J., Michonski, J., Seals, R., . . . Fonagy, P. (2009). The development of a mentalization-based outcomes and research protocol for an adolescent inpatient unit. *Bulletin of the Menninger Clinic, 73,* 311–338. http://dx.doi.org/10.1521/bumc.2009.73.4.311

Shipman, K. L., & Zeman, J. (1999). Emotional understanding: A comparison of physically maltreating and nonmaltreating mother–child dyads. *Journal of Clinical Child Psychology, 28,* 407–417. http://dx.doi.org/10.1207/S15374424jccp280313

Shmueli-Goetz, Y., Target, M., Fonagy, P., & Datta, A. (2008). The Child Attachment Interview: A psychometric study of reliability and discriminant validity. *Developmental Psychology, 44,* 939–956. http://dx.doi.org/10.1037/0012-1649.44.4.939

Siegel, D. J., & Hartzell, M. (2014). *Parenting from the inside out: How a deeper self-understanding can help you raise children who thrive.* New York, NY: Scribe.

Skårderud, F., & Fonagy, P. (2012). Eating disorders. In A. W. Bateman & P. Fonagy (Eds.), *Handbook of mentalizing in mental health practice* (pp. 347–384). Arlington, VA: American Psychiatric Publishing.

Slade, A. (1994). Making meaning and making believe: Their role in the clinical process. In A. Slade & D. Wolf (Eds.), *Children at play: Clinical and developmental approaches to meaning and representation* (pp. 81–110). Oxford, England: Oxford University Press.

Slade, A. (2005). Parental reflective functioning: An introduction. *Attachment & Human Development, 7,* 269–281. http://dx.doi.org/10.1080/14616730500245906

Slade, A. (2007). Reflective parenting programs: Theory and development. *Psychoanalytic Inquiry, 26,* 640–657. http://dx.doi.org/10.1080/07351690701310698

Slade, A. (2008). Working with parents in child psychotherapy: Engaging the reflective function. In F. N. Busch (Ed.), *Mentalization: Theoretical considerations, research findings, and clinical implications* (pp. 207–234). Mahwah, NJ: Analytic Press.

Slade, A., Aber, J. L., Bresgi, I., Berger, B., & Kaplan, M. (2004). *The Parent Development Interview—Revised.* Unpublished protocol, City University of New York, New York, NY.

Slade, A., Grienenberger, J., Bernbach, E., Levy, D., & Locker, A. (2005). Maternal reflective functioning, attachment, and the transmission gap: A preliminary study. *Attachment & Human Development*, 7, 283–298. http://dx.doi.org/10.1080/14616730500245880

Slade, A., Sadler, L., De Dios-Kenn, C., Webb, D., Currier-Ezepchick, J., & Mayes, L. (2005). Minding the baby: A reflective parenting program. *The Psychoanalytic Study of the Child*, 60, 74–100.

Slijper, F. M. E. (2008). Treatment in practice. In A. J. E. Verheugt-Pleiter, J. Zevalkink, & M. G. J. Schmeets (Eds.), *Mentalizing in child therapy: Guidelines for clinical practitioners* (pp. 179–194). London, England: Karnac Books.

Southam-Gerow, M. A., & Kendall, P. C. (2002). Emotion regulation and understanding: Implications for child psychopathology and therapy. *Clinical Psychology Review*, 22, 189–222. http://dx.doi.org/10.1016/S0272-7358(01)00087-3

Staun, L., Kessler, H., Buchheim, A., Kächele, H., & Taubner, S. (2010). Mentalisierung und chronische depression [Mentalizing and chronic depression]. *Psychotherapeut*, 55, 299–305. http://dx.doi.org/10.1007/s00278-010-0752-9

Stern, D. N. (1985). *The interpersonal world of the infant: A view from psychoanalysis and developmental psychology*. New York, NY: Basis Books.

Stern, D. N. (1992). *Diary of a baby: What your child sees, feels, and experiences*. New York, NY: Basic Books.

Stern, D. N. (2004). *The present moment in psychotherapy and everyday life*. New York, NY: Norton.

Stern, D. N. (2010). *Forms of vitality*. http://dx.doi.org/10.1093/med:psych/9780199586066.001.0001

Suchman, N. E., DeCoste, C., Leigh, D., & Borelli, J. (2010). Reflective functioning in mothers with drug use disorders: Implications for dyadic interactions with infants and toddlers. *Attachment & Human Development*, 12, 567–585. http://dx.doi.org/10.1080/14616734.2010.501988

Suchman, N. E., Pajulo, M., & Mayes, L. C. (Eds.). (2013). *Parenting and substance abuse: Developmental approaches to intervention*. New York, NY: Oxford University Press.

Svendsen, B., Tanum Johns, U., Brautaset, H., & Egebjerg, I. (2012). *Utviklingsrettet intersubjektiv psykoterapi med barn og unge [Development-oriented interpersonal psychotherapy with children and adolescents]*. Bergen, Norway: Fagbokforlaget.

Symons, D. K., Fossum, K., & Collins, T. B. K. (2006). A longitudinal study of belief and desire state discourse during mother–child play and later false belief understanding. *Social Development*, 15, 676–692. http://dx.doi.org/10.1111/j.1467-9507.2006.00364.x

Target, M., & Fonagy, P. (1996). Playing with reality: II. The development of psychic reality from a theoretical perspective. *The International Journal of Psychoanalysis*, 77, 459–479.

Target, M., Fonagy, P., & Shmueli-Goetz, Y. (2003). Attachment representations in school-age children: The development of the Child Attachment Interview

(CAI). *Journal of Child Psychotherapy, 29,* 171–186. http://dx.doi.org/10.1080/0075417031000138433

Target, M., Fonagy, P., Shmueli-Goetz, Y., Schneider, T., & Datta, A. (2000). *Child Attachment Interview (CAI): Coding and classification manual, Version III.* Unpublished manuscript, University College London, London, England.

Taumoepeau, M., & Ruffman, T. (2008). Stepping stones to others' minds: Maternal talk relates to child mental state language and emotion understanding at 15, 24, and 33 months. *Child Development, 79,* 284–302. http://dx.doi.org/10.1111/j.1467-8624.2007.01126.x

Taylor, C. (2012). *Emphatic care for children with disorganized attachments: A model for mentalizing, attachment and trauma-informed care.* London, England: Jessica Kingsley.

ten Kate, C. A., Weijers, J. G., & Smit, W. M. A. (2016). Mentaliseren bevorderende therapie voor non-affectieve psychotische stoornissen [Mentalizing-promoting therapy for nonaffective psychiatric disorders]. *PSy Expert,* 42–50.

Tessier, V. P., Normandin, L., Ensink, K., & Fonagy, P. (2016). Fact or fiction? A longitudinal study of play and the development of reflective functioning. *Bulletin of the Menninger Clinic, 80,* 60–79. http://dx.doi.org/10.1521/bumc.2016.80.1.60

Thompson, R. A., & Lagatutta, K. H. (2006). Feeling and understanding: Early emotional development. In K. McCartney & D. Phillips (Eds.), *Blackwell handbook of early childhood development* (pp. 317–337). http://dx.doi.org/10.1002/9780470757703.ch16

Thompson, R. A., Meyer, S., & McGinley, M. (2006). Understanding values in relationship: The development of conscience. In M. Killen & J. Smetana (Eds.), *Handbook of moral development* (pp. 267–297). Mahwah, NJ: Erlbaum.

Thorén, A., Pertoft Nemirovski, J., & Lindqvist, K. (2016). *Short-term mentalization-informed psychotherapy. A way of treating common childhood mental disorders.* Manuscript in preparation.

Timimi, S. (2002). *Pathological child psychiatry and the medicalization of childhood.* Hove, England: Brunner-Routledge.

Tomasello, M., & Farrar, M. J. (1986). Joint attention and early language. *Child Development, 57,* 1454–1463. http://dx.doi.org/10.2307/1130423

Trevarthen, C., Aitken, K. J., Vandekerckove, M., Delafield-Butt, J., & Nagy, E. (2006). Collaborative regulations of vitality in early childhood: Stress in intimate relationships and postnatal psychopathology. In D. Cicchetti (Ed.), *Developmental psychopathology* (Vol. 2, pp. 65–126). New York, NY: Wiley.

Tronick, E. (2007). *The neurobehavioral and social-emotional development of infants and children.* New York, NY: Norton.

Trzesniewski, K. H., Kinal, M., & Donnellan, M. B. (2010). Self-enhancement and self-protection in developmental context. In M. Alicke & C. Sedikides (Eds.), *The handbook of self-enhancement and self-protection* (pp. 341–357). New York, NY: Guilford Press.

Twemlow, S. W., Fonagy, P., & Sacco, F. C. (2005). A developmental approach to mentalizing communities: II. The Peaceful Schools experiment. *Bulletin of the Menninger Clinic, 69,* 282–304. http://dx.doi.org/10.1521/bumc.2005.69.4.282

Vaish, A., Grossmann, T., & Woodward, A. (2008). Not all emotions are created equal: The negativity bias in social-emotional development. *Psychological Bulletin, 134,* 383–403. http://dx.doi.org/10.1037/0033-2909.134.3.383

Valentino, K., Cicchetti, D., Toth, S. L., & Rogosch, F. A. (2011). Mother–child play and maltreatment: A longitudinal analysis of emerging social behavior from infancy to toddlerhood. *Developmental Psychology, 47,* 1280–1294. http://dx.doi.org/10.1037/a0024459

van IJzendoorn, M. H., & Kroonenberg, P. M. (1988). Cross-cultural patterns of attachment: A meta-analysis of the strange situation. *Child Development, 59,* 147–156. http://dx.doi.org/10.2307/1130396

Verheugt-Pleiter, A. J. (2008a). Intervention techniques: Attention regulation. In A. J. Verheugt-Pleiter, J. Zevalkink, & M. G. J. Schmeets (Eds.), *Mentalizing in child therapy* (pp. 108–131). London, England: Karnac Books.

Verheugt-Pleiter, A. J. (2008b). Treatment strategy. In A. J. Verheugt-Pleiter, J. Zevalkink, & M. G. J. Schmeets (Eds.), *Mentalizing in child therapy* (pp. 41–68). London, England: Karnac Books.

Verheugt-Pleiter, A. J., Zevalkink, J., & Schmeets, M. G. J. (Eds.). (2008). *Mentalizing in child therapy.* London, England: Karnac Books.

Vrouva, I., Target, M., & Ensink, K. (2012). Measuring mentalization in children and young people. In N. Midgley & I. Vrouva (Eds.), *Minding the child: Mentalization-based interventions with children, young people and their families* (pp. 54–77). London, England: Routledge.

Vrtička, P., Andersson, F., Grandjean, D., Sander, D., & Vuilleumier, P. (2008). Individual attachment style modulates human amygdala and striatum activation during social appraisal. *PLoS One, 3,* e2868. http://dx.doi.org/10.1371/journal.pone.0002868

Vygotsky, L. S. (1978). *Mind in society: The development of higher psychological processes.* Cambridge, MA: Harvard University Press.

Weimer, A. A., Sallquist, J., & Bolnick, R. R. (2012). Young children's emotion comprehension and theory of mind understanding. *Early Education and Development, 23,* 280–301. http://dx.doi.org/10.1080/10409289.2010.517694

Whitefield, C., & Midgley, N. (2015). "And when you were a child?" How therapists working with parents alongside individual child psychotherapy bring the past into their work. *Journal of Child Psychotherapy, 41,* 272–292. http://dx.doi.org/10.1080/0075417X.2015.1092678

Widen, S. C., & Russell, J. A. (2008). Children acquire emotion categories gradually. *Cognitive Development, 23,* 291–312. http://dx.doi.org/10.1016/j.cogdev.2008.01.002

Wieland, S., & Silberg, J. (2013). Dissociation-focused therapy. In J. D. Ford & C. A. Courtois (Eds.), *Treating complex traumatic stress disorders in children and adolescents: Scientific foundations and therapeutic models* (pp. 162–183). New York, NY: Guilford Press.

Winnicott, D. W. (1967). Mirror-role of the mother and family in child development. In P. Lomas (Ed.), *The predicament of the family: A psycho-analytical symposium* (pp. 26–33). London, England: Hogarth.

Winnicott, D. W. (1971a). *Playing and reality*. Middlesex, England: Penguin Books.

Winnicott, D. W. (1971b). *Therapeutic consultations in child psychiatry*. London, England: The Hogarth Press and the Institute of Psychoanalysis.

Winnicott, D. W. (1996). *Thinking about children*. London, England: Karnac Books.

Wood, S., Brasnett, H., Lassri, D., Fearon, P., & Midgley, N. (2015). *Mentalization based treatment for children looked after and their carers (MBT–Fostering): Treatment manual for use in the "Herts and Minds" study*. Unpublished manuscript, Anna Freud Centre/University College London, London, England.

Zevalkink, J., Verheugt-Pleiter, A., & Fonagy, P. (2012). Mentalization-informed child psychoanalytic psychotherapy. In A. W. Bateman & P. Fonagy (Eds.), *Handbook of mentalizing in mental health practice* (pp. 129–158). Arlington, VA: American Psychiatric Publishing.

INDEX

ABOUT THE AUTHORS

Nick Midgley, PhD, trained as a child and adolescent psychotherapist at the Anna Freud National Centre for Children and Families and is a senior lecturer in the Research Department of Clinical, Educational and Health Psychology at University College London. He is the codirector of the Child Attachment and Psychological Therapies Research Unit (ChAPTRe) at Anna Freud/University College London and has published widely, including coediting the book *Minding the Child: Mentalization-Based Interventions for Children, Young People and Families* (2012).

Karin Ensink, PhD, is a professor of child and adolescent psychology at the Université Laval in Québec, Canada, where she teaches mentalization-based treatment (MBT) and psychodynamic psychotherapy with children, adolescents, and parents. She completed her PhD under the direction of Mary Target and Peter Fonagy. Her research and clinical work continue to focus on the development and assessment of mentalization in children, adolescents, and parents. She has a particular interest in understanding failures of mentalization in the context of parent–child interactions and how this relates to psychopathology and personality, as well as treatment.

Karin Lindqvist, MSc, is a clinical psychologist trained in MBT for children (MBT–C) and parents at the Erica Foundation, Stockholm, Sweden, where she works part time as a researcher and clinical psychologist. Dr. Lindqvist's research concerns psychodynamic psychotherapy with children, adolescents, and adults. She is trained in reflective functioning and has done research on mentalizing capacity in clinical samples. In addition to working at the Erica Foundation, she works with children in foster placement and their families in Stockholm.

Norka Malberg, PsyD, is a certified child and adolescent psychoanalyst who trained at the Anna Freud Centre in London and obtained her doctorate at University College London for her adaptation of MBT to group work in a pediatric hospital setting. She is currently an assistant clinical professor at the Yale Child Study Center in New Haven, Connecticut, where she is also in private practice. She has a special interest in the applications of MBT to children in foster care as well as those experiencing chronic illness and other impinging somatic conditions (e.g., epilepsy, chronic eczema, asthma).

Nicole Muller, MS, MSc, is a child and adolescent psychotherapist and family therapist based at the De Jutters Child and Adolescent Mental Health Service, The Hague, Netherlands. Originally trained as a cognitive behavioral therapist, she became interested in MBT, which she has used for many years in her work with children and adolescents with attachment disorder, trauma, or emerging personality disorder and their families. One of her areas of expertise is working with fostered and adopted children and their families.